Study Guide to Accompany NASM's Essentials of Corrective Exercise Training

Author

Brian Sutton, MS, MA, PES, CES, NASM CPT

Editor

Scott Lucett MS, PES, CES, NASM CPT

Wolters Kluwer | Lippincott Williams & Wilkins
Health

Philadelphia · Baltimore · New York · London
Buenos Aires · Hong Kong · Sydney · Tokyo

Acquisitions Editor: Emily Lupash
Product Manager: Andrea Klingler
Marketing Manager: Christen Murphy
Designer: Teresa Mallon
Compositor: SPi Technologies

First Edition

Library of Congress Cataloging-in-Publication Data
ISBN: 9781608317141

DISCLAIMER

Care has been taken to confirm the accuracy of the information present and to describe generally accepted practices. However, the authors, editors, and publisher are not responsible for errors or omissions or for any consequences from application of the information in this book and make no warranty, expressed or implied, with respect to the currency, completeness, or accuracy of the contents of the publication. Application of this information in a particular situation remains the professional responsibility of the practitioner; the clinical treatments described and recommended may not be considered absolute and universal recommendations.

The authors, editors, and publisher have exerted every effort to ensure that drug selection and dosage set forth in this text are in accordance with the current recommendations and practice at the time of publication. However, in view of ongoing research, changes in government regulations, and the constant flow of information relating to drug therapy and drug reactions, the reader is urged to check the package insert for each drug for any change in indications and dosage and for added warnings and precautions. This is particularly important when the recommended agent is a new or infrequently employed drug.

Some drugs and medical devices presented in this publication have Food and Drug Administration (FDA) clearance for limited use in restricted research settings. It is the responsibility of the health care provider to ascertain the FDA status of each drug or device planned for use in their clinical practice.

To purchase additional copies of this book, call our customer service department at **(800) 638-3030** or fax orders to **(301) 223-2320**. International customers should call **(301) 223-2300**.

Visit Lippincott Williams & Wilkins on the Internet: **http://www.lww.com.** Lippincott Williams & Wilkins customer service representatives are available from 8:30 am to 6:00 pm, EST.

9 8 7 6 5 4

RRS1206

Preface

Introduction to the Course

Welcome to the National Academy of Sports Medicine (NASM) Essentials of Corrective Exercise Training. At NASM, our mission is to help provide health and fitness professionals with the best evidence-based education and systems. Our educational continuum employs an easy-to-use, systematic approach in order to apply scientific, clinically accepted concepts.

The NASM Essentials of Corrective Exercise Training was developed in response to the growing need for professionals to successfully assist clients experiencing musculoskeletal impairments, muscle imbalances, or rehabilitation concerns. By gaining advanced injury prevention and recovery knowledge, you place yourself on a career path that leads to professional success through expansive professional capabilities, increased revenue generating potential through untapped markets, as well as reaching a benchmark of educational excellence in the health and fitness industry.

How to Use This Study Guide

The purpose of this study guide is to help you master the basic concepts presented in the text. This study guide provides students with a way to evaluate their knowledge, strengths, and weaknesses through an interactive review process.

Study Tips

The most important characteristic for students to possess is a deep and passionate desire to learn. That said, the following tips should help maximize the time spent on the course materials:

1. *Pace yourself.* Allow yourself enough time to get through the materials and thoroughly comprehend the information before progressing within the course.

2. *Schedule your study time.* This will ensure a reasonable timeframe for completing your work.

3. *Read and re-read.* When reviewing the course text, scan the information once to obtain an overview of the material. Then, go back and read the information thoroughly.

4. *Think about it.* Stop frequently as you review course material to consider the concepts presented. Ask yourself how and when you can apply the techniques and information covered.

5. *Lighten up.* Use a highlighter to accent important concepts and information or areas that may require additional review and practice.

6. *Do the exercises.* NASM strongly recommends going through the exercises for each section after you have completed your reading.

7. *Practice, practice, practice.* Remember that regular review and application of these principles is essential to your success. Apply what you've learned at every opportunity to help improve your techniques.

Getting Help

At NASM, your success is our success. We want to help in every way we can. The NASM staff is available to offer any assistance you may need throughout the course of your program. Whether you have technical or educational questions, we are available by phone and email 8:00 AM to 5:00 PM (PST), Monday through Friday. Please call our toll-free number at 800.460. NASM or log onto our website *www.nasm.org* to email us questions.

Contents

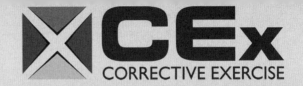

INTRODUCTION TO CORRECTIVE EXERCISE TRAINING

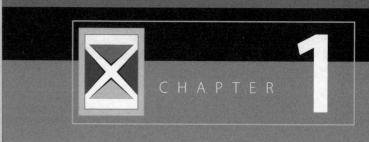

70-75% of ACL injuries are non-contact in nature.

shoulder pain for 21%.

80,000 to 100,000 ACL injuries annually

CHAPTER 1

T[...] for C[...]ercises

EXERCISE 1-1 **Essential Vocabulary**

PURPOSE: The purpose of this exercise is to have an understanding of key terms used in Chapter 1.

INSTRUCTIONS: Match each term with its proper definition.

VOCABULARY WORDS

1. ___ Corrective exercise

2. ___ The Corrective Exercise Continuum

3. ___ Inhibitory techniques

4. ___ Lengthening techniques

5. ___ Activation techniques

6. ___ Integration techniques

DEFINITIONS

A. Corrective exercise techniques used to release tension or decrease activity of overactive neuromyofascial tissues in the body.

B. Corrective exercise techniques used to increase the extensibility, length, and range of motion of neuromyofascial tissues in the body.

C. Corrective exercise techniques used to retrain the collective synergistic function of all muscles through functionally progressive movements.

D. The systematic programming process used to address neuromusculoskeletal dysfunction through the use of inhibitory, lengthening, activation, and integration techniques.

E. Corrective exercise techniques used to reeducate or increase activation of underactive tissues.

F. A term used to describe the systematic process of identifying a neuromusculoskeletal dysfunction, developing a plan of action, and implementing an integrated corrective strategy.

EXERCISE 1-2   True/False

INSTRUCTIONS: Choose whether each statement is true or false.

1. In 1985 the International Obesity Task Force deemed the prevalence of obesity an epidemic.
   True   False

2. Today, approximately one sixth (16%) of adults are estimated to be obese.
   True   False

3. Eighteen percent of today's adolescents and teenagers are considered overweight.
   True   False

4. Research suggests that musculoskeletal pain is less common now than it was 40 years ago because of the advancements of technology and manual-labor–saving devices.
   True   False

5. In the general population, plantar fasciitis accounts for more than 1 million ambulatory care (doctor) visits per year.
   True   False

6. More than one third of all work-related injuries involve the trunk, and of these, more than 60% involve the low back.
   True   False

7. It has been estimated that the annual costs attributable to low-back pain in the United States are greater than $26 billion.
   True   False

8. Approximately 20 to 25% of ACL injuries are noncontact in nature.
   True   False

9. Shoulder pain is reported to occur in up to 21% of the general population.
   True   False

10. The less conditioned our musculoskeletal systems are, the higher the risk of injury.
    True   False

EXERCISE 1-3   Multiple Choice

INSTRUCTIONS: Select the best answer from the choices given for each question.

1. _____ are reported to be the most common sports-related injury.
   a. Ankle sprains
   b. Shoulder dislocations
   c. ACL tears
   d. Head trauma

2. Individuals who suffer a lateral ankle sprain are at risk for developing:
    a. diabetic neuropathy.
    b. chronic ankle instability.
    c. pes cavus.
    d. athlete's foot.

3. Low-back pain is one of the major forms of musculoskeletal degeneration seen in the adult population, affecting nearly:
    a. 20% of all adults.
    b. 40% of all adults.
    c. 60% of all adults.
    d. 80% of all adults.

4. An estimated _____ anterior cruciate ligament (ACL) injuries occur annually in the general U.S. population.
    a. 8,000 to 10,000
    b. 20,000 to 40,000
    c. 80,000 to 100,000
    d. 200,000 to 300,000

5. What is the most prevalent diagnosis of shoulder pain?
    a. Shoulder impingement
    b. Shoulder dislocation
    c. Rotator cuff tear
    d. Frozen shoulder

6. Most ACL injuries occur between:
    a. 15 and 25 years of age.
    b. 30 and 40 years of age.
    c. 55 and 65 years of age.
    d. 70 and 80 years of age.

7. According to the text, a comprehensive corrective exercise strategy using the Corrective Exercise Continuum includes all of the following steps EXCEPT:
    a. Identify the problem (integrated assessment)
    b. Solve the problem (corrective program design)
    c. Implement the solution (exercise technique)
    d. R.I.C.E. (rest, ice, compress, elevate)

8. What is the correct order of the Corrective Exercise Continuum?
    a. Inhibit → Lengthen → Activate → Integrate
    b. Lengthen → Inhibit → Integrate → Activate
    c. Activate → Integrate → Lengthen → Inhibit
    d. Integrate → Activate → Lengthen → Inhibit

9. Which phase of the Corrective Exercise Continuum uses self-myofascial release techniques to decrease activity of overactive neuromyofascial tissues in the body?
    a. Lengthen
    b. Inhibit
    c. Activate
    d. Integrate

10. Which phase of the Corrective Exercise Continuum uses isolated strengthening exercises and positional isometric techniques?
    a. Inhibit
    b. Lengthen
    c. Activate
    d. Integrate

CHAPTER 2

Introduction to Human Movement Science

EXERCISE 2-1   Essential Vocabulary

PURPOSE: The purpose of this exercise is to have an understanding of key terms used in Chapter 2.

INSTRUCTIONS: Match each term with its proper definition.

VOCABULARY WORDS

1. ___ Biomechanics

2. ___ Force

3. ___ Rotary motion

4. ___ Torque

5. ___ Agonist

6. ___ Antagonists

7. ___ Synergists

8. ___ Stabilizers

9. ___ Motor behavior

10. ___ Motor control

11. ___ Motor learning

12. ___ Motor development

13. ___ Internal (sensory) feedback

14. ___ External (augmented) feedback

DEFINITIONS

A. Movement of the bones around the joints.

B. Muscles that assist prime movers during functional movement patterns.

C. Muscles that act as prime movers.

D. A force that produces rotation.

E. A study that uses principles of physics to quantitatively study how forces interact within a living body.

F. Information provided by some external source, for example, a health and fitness professional, videotape, mirror, or heart rate monitor.

G. An influence applied by one object to another, which results in an acceleration or deceleration of the second object.

H. Muscles that act in direct opposition to prime movers.

I. Feedback used after the completion of a movement to help inform the client about the outcome of his or her performance.

15. ___ Knowledge of results

16. ___ Knowledge of performance

17. ___ Length-tension relationship

18. ___ Force-velocity curve

19. ___ Force-couple

20. ___ Local musculature system

21. ___ Global musculature system

22. ___ Sensory information

23. ___ Sensation

24. ___ Perception

25. ___ Sensorimotor integration

26. ___ Feedback

J. The change in motor behavior with time throughout the lifespan.

K. Integration of motor control processes through practice and experience leading to a relatively permanent change in the capacity to produce skilled movements.

L. The human movement system's response to internal and external environmental stimuli.

M. Muscles that support or stabilize the body while the prime movers and the synergists perform the movement patterns.

N. The process by which sensory information is used by the body via length-tension relationships, force-couple relationships, and arthrokinematics to monitor movement and the environment.

O. The study of posture and movements with the involved structures and mechanisms used by the central nervous system to assimilate and integrate sensory information with previous experiences.

P. Feedback that provides information about the quality of the movement during exercise.

Q. The utilization of sensory information · and sensorimotor integration to aid in the development of permanent neural representations of motor patterns for efficient movement.

R. The integration of sensory information with past experiences or memories.

S. A process whereby sensory information is received by the receptor and transferred either to the spinal cord for reflexive motor behavior or to higher cortical areas for processing, or both.

T. The data that the central nervous system receives from sensory receptors to determine such things as the body's position in space and limb orientation, as well as information about the environment, temperature, texture, and so forth.

U. Muscles responsible predominantly for movement, consisting of more superficial musculature that originates from the pelvis to the rib cage, the lower extremities, or both.

[Handwritten answers:]

```
1 E     14 F
2 G     15 I
3 A     16 P          14
4 Z D   17 Y Z        ——
5 C     18 B Y        26
6 H     19 V
7 B     20 M W
8 W M   21 U
9 Q L   22 L T
10 X O  23 F S
11 K    24 R
12 J    25 N X
13 N    26 S Q
```

V. The synergistic action of muscles to produce movement around a joint.

W. Muscles that are predominantly involved in joint support or stabilization.

X. The ability of the central nervous system to gather and interpret sensory information to execute the proper motor response.

Y. The relationship of muscle's ability to produce tension at differing shortening velocities.

Z. The resting length of a muscle and the tension the muscle can produce at this resting length.

EXERCISE 2-2   Knowledge of Terms

INSTRUCTIONS: Use the following terms to fill in the blanks below.

Transverse plane   Pronation
Sagittal plane   Supination
Concentric contraction   Isometric contraction
Frontal plane   Eccentric contraction

[Handwritten answers:]

```
2-2
1 sagital plane
2 frontal plane
3 transverse plane
4 pronation contraction
5 supination contraction
6 eccentric ... at
7 isometric contraction
8 concentric ... action
```

1. _____ bisects the body into right and left halves, and ...es flexion and extension movements.

2. _____ bisects the body into front and back halves, ...cludes abduction and adduction of the limbs (relative to the ...exion of the spine, and eversion and inversion of the foot and

3. _____ bisects the body to create upper and lower ...arily includes internal rotation and external rotation for the ...left rotation for the head and trunk, and radioulnar pronation

4. _____ is a multiplanar, synchronized joint motion that ...ntric muscle function.

5. _____ is a multiplanar, synchronized joint motion that occurs with concentric muscle function.

6. An _____ occurs when a muscle develops tension while lengthening.

7. An _____ occurs when the contractile force is equal to the resistive force, leading to no visible change in the muscle length.

8. A _____ occurs when the contractile force is greater than the resistive force, resulting in shortening of the muscle and visible joint movement.

EXERCISE 2-3   Multiple Choice

INSTRUCTIONS: Select the best answer from the choices given for each question.

1. What are the major muscle groups of the lateral sub-system?
   a. Gluteus medius, tensor fascia latae, adductor complex, quadratus lomborum
   b. Anterior tibialis, posterior tibialis, erector spinae, posterior deltoid
   c. Pectoralis major, rhomboids, trapezius, adductor complex
   d. Rectus abdominis, external oblique, internal oblique

2. What are the major muscle groups of the deep longitudinal sub-system?
   a. Pectoralis major, pectoralis minor, triceps brachii
   b. Erector spinae, thoracolumbar fascia, sacrotuberous ligament, biceps femoris, peroneus longus
   c. Upper, middle, and lower trapezius
   d. Gastrocnemius, soleus, peroneus longus, peroneus brevis

3. What are the major muscle groups of the anterior oblique sub-system?
   a. Gluteus maximus, gluteus medius, gluteus minimus
   b. Quadriceps, hamstring complex, gluteus maximus
   c. Internal and external obliques, adductor complex, hip external rotators
   d. Multifidus, diaphragm, erector spinae, psoas

4. Which sub-system works synergistically with the deep longitudinal sub-system and consists of the gluteus maximus, thoracolumbar fascia, and contralateral latissimus dorsi?
   a. Deep longitudinal sub-system
   b. Anterior oblique sub-system
   c. Lateral sub-system
   d. Posterior oblique sub-system

5. The joint support system of the lumbo-pelvic-hip complex (LPHC) includes the following muscles.
   a. Transverse abdominis, multifidus, internal oblique, diaphragm, pelvic floor muscles
   b. Rectus abdominis, external oblique, latissimus dorsi
   c. Rectus femoris, biceps femoris, psoas
   d. Pectoralis minor, erector spinae, levator scapulae, sternocleidomastoid

6. What is the cumulative neural input from sensory afferents to the central nervous system?
   a. Sensation
   b. Perception
   c. Proprioception
   d. Force-couple relationships

7. What part of the nervous system is designed to optimize muscle synergies?
   a. Peripheral
   b. Autonomic
   c. Parasympathetic
   d. Central

8. Flexion at the ankle is more accurately termed what?

   a. Dorsiflexion
   b. Plantar flexion
   c. Eversion
   d. Inversion

9. What is the concentric function of the anterior tibialis?

   a. Accelerates ankle plantar flexion and inversion
   b. Accelerates ankle dorsiflexion and eversion
   c. Accelerates ankle dorsiflexion and inversion
   d. Accelerates ankle plantar flexion and eversion

10. What is the eccentric function of the gluteus medius (posterior fibers)?

    a. Decelerates hip adduction and internal rotation
    b. Decelerates hip abduction and internal rotation
    c. Decelerates hip abduction and external rotation
    d. Decelerates hip adduction and external rotation

11. What is the concentric function of the latissimus dorsi?

    a. Shoulder flexion, abduction, and external rotation
    b. Shoulder extension, abduction, and external rotation
    c. Shoulder flexion, adduction, and internal rotation
    d. Shoulder extension, adduction, and internal rotation

12. What is the concentric function of the posterior tibialis?

    a. Accelerates ankle plantar flexion and inversion
    b. Accelerates ankle dorsiflexion and eversion
    c. Accelerates ankle dorsiflexion and inversion
    d. Accelerates ankle plantar flexion and eversion

13. What is the concentric function of the biceps femoris (short head)?

    a. Accelerates knee flexion and tibial internal rotation
    b. Accelerates knee extension and tibial internal rotation
    c. Accelerates knee flexion and tibial external rotation
    d. Accelerates knee extension and tibial external rotation

14. What is the concentric function of tensor fascia latae?

    a. Accelerates hip flexion, abduction, and internal rotation
    b. Accelerates hip extension, adduction, and internal rotation
    c. Accelerates hip extension, abduction, and external rotation
    d. Accelerates hip flexion, adduction, and external rotation

15. What is the eccentric function of the pectoralis major?

    a. Shoulder flexion, horizontal adduction, and external rotation
    b. Shoulder extension, horizontal abduction, and external rotation
    c. Shoulder flexion, horizontal abduction, and internal rotation
    d. Shoulder extension, horizontal adduction, and internal rotation

1. a
2. b
3. c
4. ed
5. ea
6. AC
7. bd
8. a

9. c
10. a
11. d
12. ea
13. c
14. a
15. B

CHAPTER 3

An Evidence-Based Approach to Understanding Human Movement Impairments

EXERCISE 3-1   **Essential Vocabulary**

PURPOSE: The purpose of this exercise is to have an understanding of key terms used in Chapter 3.

INSTRUCTIONS: Match each term with its proper definition.

VOCABULARY WORDS

1. ___ Neuromuscular efficiency

2. ___ Posture

3. ___ Structural efficiency

4. ___ Functional efficiency

5. ___ Cumulative injury cycle

6. ___ Movement impairment syndrome

7. ___ Altered reciprocal inhibition

8. ___ Synergistic dominance

9. ___ Lower extremity movement impairment syndrome

10. ___ Upper extremity movement impairment syndrome

DEFINITIONS

A. The alignment of each segment of the human movement system (HMS), which allows posture to be balanced in relation to one's center of gravity.

B. The process whereby a tight muscle (short, overactive, myofascial adhesions) causes decreased neural drive, and therefore optimal recruitment of its functional antagonist.

C. Usually characterized as having rounded shoulders and a forward head posture or improper scapulothoracic or glenohumeral kinematics during functional movements.

D. The independent and interdependent alignment (static posture) and function (transitional and dynamic posture) of all components of the human movement system at any given moment; controlled by the central nervous system.

E. The process by which a synergist compensates for a prime mover to maintain force production.

F. A cycle in which an injury will induce inflammation, muscle spasm, adhesion, altered neuromuscular control, and muscle imbalances.

G. The ability of the neuromuscular system to allow agonists, antagonists, synergists, and stabilizers to work synergistically to produce, reduce, and dynamically stabilize the kinetic chain in all three planes of motion.

H. Refers to the state in which the structural integrity of the human movement system (HMS) is compromised because the components are out of alignment.

I. Usually characterized by excessive foot pronation (flat feet), increased knee valgus (tibia externally rotated and femur internally rotated and adducted or knock-kneed), and increased movement at the lumbo-pelvic-hip complex (extension or flexion) during functional movements.

J. The ability of the neuromuscular system to recruit correct muscle synergies, at the right time, with the appropriate amount of force to perform functional tasks with the least amount of energy and stress on the human movement system.

EXERCISE 3-2　True/False

INSTRUCTIONS: Choose whether each statement is true or false.

1. Because the human movement system is an integrated system, impairment in one system leads to compensations and adaptations in other systems.
   True　False

2. If one segment in the human movement system is out of alignment, then other movement segments have to compensate in attempts to balance the weight distribution of the dysfunctional segment.
   True　False

3. If the gluteus medius is underactive, then the tensor fascia latae (TFL) may become synergistically dominant to produce the necessary force to accomplish frontal plane stability of the lumbo-pelvic-hip complex.
   True　False

4. Once a joint has lost its normal arthrokinematics, the muscles around that joint may spasm in an attempt to minimize the stress at the involved segment.
   True　False

5. Synergistic dominance is the process by which a tight muscle causes decreased neural drive of its functional antagonist.
   True　False

6. A tight psoas decreasing the neural drive and optimal recruitment of the gluteus maximus is an example of synergistic dominance.

   True   False

7. If a client has a weak gluteus medius, then synergists (tensor fascia latae, adductor complex, and quadratus lumborum) oftentimes become synergistically dominant to compensate for the weakness.

   True   False

8. Individuals with a lower extremity movement impairment syndrome are usually characterized by excessive foot pronation (flat feet), increased knee valgus (knock-kneed), and increased movement at the lumbo-pelvic-hip complex (extension or flexion) during functional movements.

   True   False

9. Individuals with the upper extremity movement impairment syndrome are usually characterized as having rounded shoulders and a forward head posture or improper scapulothoracic or glenohumeral kinematics during functional movements.

   True   False

10. Individuals who present with the lower extremity movement impairment syndrome typically develop predictable patterns of injury including rotator cuff impingement, shoulder instability, biceps tendinitis, thoracic outlet syndrome, and headaches.

    True   False

EXERCISE 3-3   Multiple Choice

INSTRUCTIONS: Select the best answer from the choices given for each question.

1. It is hypothesized that decreased posterior glide of the ___ can decrease ___ at the ankle.

   a. talus, dorsiflexion
   b. phalanges, dorsiflexion
   c. cuboid, pronation
   d. metatarsals, plantar flexion

2. Most knee injuries occur during noncontact ___ in the frontal and ___ plane.

   a. acceleration, transverse
   b. acceleration, sagittal
   c. deceleration, sagittal
   d. deceleration, transverse

3. Abnormal contraction intensity and onset timing of the _____ and _____ have been demonstrated in subjects with patellofemoral pain (PFP).

   a. vastus medialis oblique, vastus lateralis
   b. tensor fascia latae, psoas minor
   c. anterior cruciate ligament, biceps femoris
   d. superficial erector spinae, piriformis

4. Potentially tightened or overactive muscles accompanying a lower extremity movement impairment syndrome include the following EXCEPT:

   a. peroneals.
   b. soleus.
   c. lateral gastrocnemius.
   d. anterior tibialis.

5. Potentially weakened or inhibited muscles accompanying a lower extremity movement impairment syndrome include the following EXCEPT:

   a. posterior tibialis.
   b. anterior tibialis.
   c. iliotibial band.
   d. pes anserine complex.

6. Potentially tightened or overactive muscles accompanying an upper extremity movement impairment syndrome include the following EXCEPT:

   a. pectoralis major.
   b. rhomboids.
   c. anterior deltoid.
   d. latissimus dorsi.

7. Potentially weakened or inhibited muscles accompanying an upper extremity movement impairment syndrome include the following EXCEPT:

   a. lower trapezius.
   b. teres minor.
   c. infraspinatus.
   d. sternocleidomastoid.

8. According to research, subjects demonstrating increased dynamic knee valgus typically exhibit all of the following EXCEPT:

   a. increased adductor activity.
   b. increased gluteus medius activity.
   c. decreased dorsiflexion.
   d. decreased neuromuscular control of the core.

9. Subjects with low-back pain (LBP) have been reported to demonstrate impaired postural control, delayed muscle relaxation, and abnormal muscle recruitment patterns (diminished activation) of the

   a. transverse abdominis and multifidus.
   b. rectus abdominis and external oblique.
   c. tensor fascia latae and psoas.
   d. latissimus dorsi and piriformis.

10. Which muscles are lengthened, altering the normal scapulothoracic force-couple relationship when an individual exhibits a rounded shoulder posture?

    a. Rhomboids, lower trapezius
    b. Serratus anterior, pectoralis minor
    c. Latissimus dorsi, anterior deltoid
    d. Pectoralis major, coracobrachialis

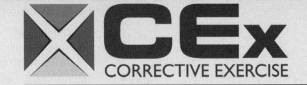
CORRECTIVE EXERCISE

ASSESSING FOR HUMAN MOVEMENT DYSFUNCTION

CHAPTER 4

Health Risk Appraisal

EXERCISE 4-1   Short Answer

1. What are the three main pieces of information a health and fitness professional should obtain from the health risk appraisal?

   _____

   _____

   _____

   _____

2. What is the purpose and function of the Physical Activity Readiness Questionnaire?

   _____

   _____

   _____

   _____

3. Briefly explain how sitting for extended periods of time has an impact on the human movement system?

   _____

   _____

   _____

   _____

4. From a human movement system standpoint, briefly describe how construction workers and painters can develop muscle imbalances and injury of the upper extremities.

   _____

   _____

   _____

   _____

5. Briefly describe how wearing shoes with an elevated heel (dress shoes, high heels) can have an impact on the human movement system.

_____

_____

_____

_____

EXERCISE 4-2   True/False

INSTRUCTIONS: Choose whether each statement is true or false.

1. Mental stress or anxiety can lead to a dysfunctional breathing pattern that can further lead to postural distortion and kinetic chain dysfunction.

   True   False

2. Questions pertaining to an individual's recreational activities and hobbies are not an essential component of the health risk appraisal.

   True   False

3. One of the best predictors of future injuries is past injury.

   True   False

4. Ankle sprains have been shown to decrease the neural control to the gluteus medius and gluteus maximus muscles.

   True   False

5. Knee injury can cause a decrease in the neural control to muscles that stabilize the patellofemoral and tibiofemoral joints and lead to further injury.

   True   False

6. Low-back injuries can cause decreased neural control to stabilizing muscles of the core, resulting in poor stabilization of the spine and possible further dysfunction of the upper or lower extremities.

   True   False

7. Surgery will cause pain and inflammation that can alter neural control to the affected muscles and joints if not rehabilitated properly.

   True   False

8. It is estimated that roughly 25% of the American adult population does not partake, on a daily basis, in 30 minutes of low-to-moderate physical activity.

   True   False

9. One of the roles of a health and fitness professional (i.e., personal trainer, athletic trainer, strength coach) is to administer, prescribe, and educate on the usage and effects of common medications.

   True   False

10. At best, an individual/client can recall only half his or her injury history, so a close examination of imbalances through further assessments can turn up additional areas of potential risks.

    True   False

EXERCISE 4-3   **Practical Application**

Below are answers to a client's health risk appraisal. What are some potential "red flags" that may need to be considered when designing a corrective exercise program?

_____

_____

_____

_____

NAME: _____ John Doe _____   DATE: 2/17/10 _____

HEIGHT: 5'10" _____   WEIGHT: 175 lb _____   AGE: 33 _____

PHYSICIAN'S NAME: _____ Dr. Smith _____   PHONE: 555-555-1234 _____

PHYSICAL ACTIVITY READINESS QUESTIONNAIRE (PAR-Q)		
Questions	**Yes**	**No**
1. Has your doctor ever said that you have a heart condition and that you should only perform physical activity recommended by a doctor?		√
2. Do you feel pain in your chest when you perform physical activity?		√
3. During the past month, have you had chest pain when you were not performing any physical activity?		√
4. Do you lose your balance because of dizziness or do you ever lose consciousness?		√
5. Do you have a bone or joint problem that could be made worse by a change in your physical activity?		√
6. Is your doctor currently prescribing any medication for your blood pressure or for a heart condition?		√
7. Do you know of any other reason why you should not engage in physical		√

If you have answered "Yes" to one or more of the above questions, consult your physician before engaging in physical activity. Tell your physician which questions you answered "Yes" to. After a medical evaluation, seek advice from your physician on what type of activity is suitable for your current condition.

GENERAL AND MEDICAL QUESTIONNAIRE		
Occupational Questions	**Yes**	**No**
1. What is your current occupation? Computer programmer		
2. Does your occupation require extended periods of sitting?	√	
3. Does your occupation require extended periods of repetitive movements? (If yes, please explain.)		√
4. Does your occupation require you to wear shoes with a heel (dress shoes)?	√	
5. Does your occupation cause you anxiety (mental stress)?	√	

	Recreational Questions	Yes	No
6	Do you partake in any recreational activities (golf, tennis, skiing, etc.)? (If yes, please explain.) _____ _____ _____		√
7	Do you have any hobbies (reading, gardening, working on cars, exploring the Internet, etc.)? (If yes, please explain.) Reading and playing video games	√	

	Medical Questions	Yes	No
8	Have you ever had any pain or injuries (ankle, knee, hip, back, shoulder, etc.)? (If yes, please explain.) Intermittent low back pain _____ _____ _____	√	
9	Have you ever had any surgeries? (If yes, please explain.) _____ _____ _____		√
10	Has a medical doctor ever diagnosed you with a chronic disease, such as coronary heart disease, coronary artery disease, hypertension (high blood pressure), high cholesterol or diabetes? (If yes, please explain.) _____ _____ _____		√
11	Are you currently taking any medication? (If yes, please list.) _____ _____ _____		√

CHAPTER 5

Static Postural Assessments

EXERCISE 5-1   Essential Vocabulary

PURPOSE: The purpose of this exercise is to have an understanding of key terms used in Chapter 5.

INSTRUCTIONS: Match each term with its proper definition.

VOCABULARY WORDS

1. ___ Static posture

2. ___ Dynamic posture

3. ___ Hypomobility

4. ___ Myofascial

5. ___ Muscle imbalance

6. ___ Coordination

7. ___ Lower crossed syndrome

8. ___ Upper crossed syndrome

9. ___ Pronation distortion syndrome

DEFINITIONS

A. How an individual is able to maintain an erect posture while performing functional tasks.

B. The rate of muscle recruitment and the timing of muscular contractions within the kinetic chain.

C. The connective tissue in and around muscles and tendons.

D. A dysfunctional muscle pattern characterized by an anterior tilt to the pelvis and lower extremity muscle imbalances.

E. How individuals physically present themselves in stance.

F. A dysfunctional muscle pattern characterized by a forward head and rounded shoulders with upper extremity muscle imbalances.

G. Restricted motion.

H. A dysfunctional muscle pattern characterized by foot pronation and lower extremity muscle imbalances.

I. Alteration in the functional relationship between pairs or groups of muscles.

EXERCISE 5-2 True/False

INSTRUCTIONS: Choose whether each statement is true or false.

1. A static postural assessment provides indicators of problem areas that must be further evaluated to clarify the problems at hand.

   True   False

2. Treating symptomatic complaints using anti-inflammatory medications, modification of activities, or simply pushing through the pain may lead to further dysfunction, adding layer on layer of structural and neuromuscular adaptations.

   True   False

3. Looking for causative factors (versus treating symptomatic complaints) of inflammation, discomfort, or poor performance will likely result in the selection of effective intervention strategies to alleviate the dysfunction.

   True   False

4. A static postural assessment can accurately identify whether a problem is structural (or biomechanical) in nature or is derived from the development of poor muscular recruitment patterns with resultant muscle imbalances.

   True   False

5. There may be several causative factors for changes in joint alignment including quality and function of myofascial tissue and alterations in muscle-tendon function.

   True   False

6. The combination of tight and weak muscles typically does not alter normal movement patterns.

   True   False

7. Work (computer) stations both at home and at the office frequently contribute to neck and arm dysfunction.

   True   False

8. Muscle that is repeatedly placed in a shortened position, such as the iliopsoas complex during sitting, will eventually adapt and tend to remain short.

   True   False

9. Chronic use of the right lower extremity while driving, without awareness of trying to maintain symmetry, may allow the body to shift to the right and promote external rotation of the left lower extremity.

   True   False

10. Immobilizations through splinting or self-immobilization as a result of pain may allow tissue to tighten.

    True   False

EXERCISE 5-3   Multiple Choice

INSTRUCTIONS: Select the best answer from the choices given for each question.

1. According to the text, which of the following muscles is prone to lengthening (weakness)?

   a. Gastrocnemius
   b. Adductors
   c. Psoas
   d. Vastus medialis oblique

2. According to the text, which of the following muscles is prone to tightness?

   a. Anterior tibialis
   b. Rhomboids
   c. Pectoralis major/minor
   d. Gluteus maximus

3. All of the following are potential factors that cause postural imbalance EXCEPT:

   a. altered movement patterns from repetitive movement.
   b. altered movement patterns from injury.
   c. habitual movement patterns.
   d. static stretching of overactive tissues before competition.

4. Which postural distortion pattern is characterized by increased lumbar lordosis and an anterior pelvic tilt?

   a. Lower crossed syndrome
   b. Upper crossed syndrome
   c. Pronation distortion syndrome
   d. Thoracic outlet syndrome

5. Which postural distortion pattern is characterized by rounded shoulders and a forward head posture?

   a. Pronation distortion syndrome
   b. Upper crossed syndrome
   c. Thoracic outlet syndrome
   d. Lower crossed syndrome

6. Which postural distortion pattern is characterized by excessive foot pronation (flat feet), knee flexion, internal rotation, and adduction (knock-kneed)?

   a. Pronation distortion syndrome
   b. Upper crossed syndrome
   c. Thoracic outlet syndrome
   d. Lower crossed syndrome

INSTRUCTIONS: Refer to the images and then answer the questions below.

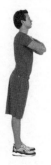

7. Which postural distortion pattern is demonstrated in the image above?
    a. Pronation distortion syndrome
    b. Upper crossed syndrome
    c. Thoracic outlet syndrome
    d. Lower crossed syndrome

8. All of the following muscles are MOST likely tight (overactive) EXCEPT the:
    a. gastrocnemius.
    b. erector spinae.
    c. adductor complex.
    d. posterior tibialis.

9. All of the following muscles are MOST likely weak (underactive) EXCEPT the:
    a. anterior tibialis.
    b. gluteus medius.
    c. hip flexor complex.
    d. transverse abdominus.

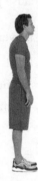

10. Which postural distortion pattern is demonstrated in the image above?
    a. Pronation distortion syndrome
    b. Upper crossed syndrome
    c. Thoracic outlet syndrome
    d. Lower Crossed syndrome

11. All of the following muscles are typically tight when an individual exhibits this postural distortion pattern EXCEPT the:
    a. pectoralis major.
    b. latissimus dorsi.
    c. subscapularis.
    d. teres minor.

12. All of the following muscles are typically weak when an individual exhibits this postural distortion pattern EXCEPT the:

    a. lower trapezius.
    b. rhomboids.
    c. scalenes.
    d. infraspinatus.

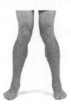

13. Which postural distortion pattern is demonstrated in the image above?

    a. Pronation distortion syndrome
    b. Upper crossed syndrome
    c. Thoracic outlet syndrome
    d. Lower crossed syndrome

14. Functionally weakened (inhibited) muscles associated with this postural distortion pattern include all of the following EXCEPT the:

    a. soleus.
    b. gluteus maximus.
    c. posterior tibialis.
    d. anterior tibialis.

15. Functionally tightened muscles associated with this postural distortion pattern include all of the following EXCEPT the:

    a. IT-band.
    b. hamstring complex.
    c. psoas.
    d. hip external rotators.

CHAPTER 6

Movement Assessments

EXERCISE 6-1   ## Essential Vocabulary

PURPOSE: The purpose of this exercise is to have an understanding of key terms used in Chapter 6.

INSTRUCTIONS: Match each term with its proper definition.

VOCABULARY WORDS

1. ___ Muscle balance

2. ___ Kinetic chain

3. ___ Transitional movement assessment

4. ___ Dynamic movement assessment

5. ___ Balance threshold

DEFINITIONS

A. Assessments that involve movement without a change in one's base of support.

B. The distance one can squat down on one leg while keeping the knee aligned in a neutral position (in line with the second and third toes).

C. The force transference from the nervous system to the muscular and skeletal systems as well as from joint to joint, which are interconnected in the body.

D. Establishing normal length-tension relationships, which ensures proper length and strength of each muscle around a joint.

E. Assessments that involve movement with a change in one's base of support.

EXERCISE 6-2   True/False

INSTRUCTIONS: Choose whether each statement is true or false.

1. Muscle balance is essential for optimal recruitment of force-couples to maintain precise joint motion and ultimately decrease excessive stress placed on the body.
   True   False

2. Any muscle, whether in a shortened or lengthened state, can be underactive or weak because of altered length-tension relationships or altered reciprocal inhibition.
   True   False

3. Alterations in muscle activity will change the biomechanical motion of the joint and lead to increased stress on the tissues of the joint and eventual injury.
   True   False

4. Movement assessments can be categorized into two types: transitional assessments and dynamic assessments.
   True   False

5. Transitional movement assessments are assessments that involve movement with a change in one's base of support such as walking and jumping.
   True   False

6. Dynamic movement assessments are assessments that involve movement without a change in one's base of support such as squatting, pressing, pushing, pulling, and balancing.
   True   False

7. Knee valgus during the overhead squat test is influenced by decreased hip adductor and hip internal rotation strength, increased hip abductor activity, and restricted ankle plantar flexion.
   True   False

8. If an individual's knees move inward during the overhead squat assessment, but the compensation is then corrected after elevating the heels, the primary region that mostly likely needs to be addressed is the foot and ankle complex.
   True   False

9. If an individual's low back arches during the overhead squat assessment, but the compensation is then corrected when performing the squat with hands on hips, the primary regions that most likely need to be addressed are the latissimus dorsi and pectoral muscles.
   True   False

10. The single-leg squat assessment assesses dynamic flexibility, core strength, balance, and overall neuromuscular control.
    True   False

EXERCISE 6-3   Multiple Choice

INSTRUCTIONS: Review the image then answer the following questions.

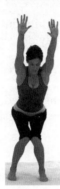

1. What is the *primary* movement compensation demonstrated during the overhead squat assessment?
   a. Arms fall forward
   b. Knees move inward
   c. Low back arches
   d. Excessive forward lean

2. Which muscle is *most* likely overactive?
   a. Medial hamstring complex
   b. Medial gastrocnemius
   c. Adductor complex
   d. Gluteus medius

3. Which muscle is *most* likely underactive?
   a. Gluteus medius
   b. Tensor fascia latae
   c. Adductor complex
   d. Biceps femoris (short head)

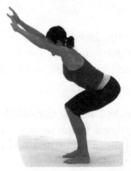

4. What is the *primary* movement compensation demonstrated during the overhead squat assessment?
   a. Arms fall forward
   b. Low back rounds
   c. Low back arches
   d. Excessive forward lean

5. Which muscle is *most* likely overactive?

    a. Hip flexor complex
    b. Erector spinae
    c. Anterior tibialis
    d. Gluteus maximus

6. Which muscle is *most* likely underactive?

    a. Gastrocnemius
    b. Soleus
    c. Hip flexor complex
    d. Gluteus maximus

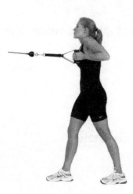

7. What is the *primary* movement compensation demonstrated during the pulling assessment?

    a. Shoulders elevate
    b. Low back arches
    c. Low back rounds
    d. Excessive forward lean

8. Which muscle is *most* likely overactive?

    a. Rotator cuff
    b. Upper trapezius
    c. Lower trapezius
    d. Rhomboids

9. Which muscle is *most* likely underactive?

    a. Lower trapezius
    b. Upper trapezius
    c. Sternocleidomastoid
    d. Levator scapulae

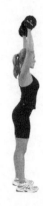

10. What is the *primary* movement compensation demonstrated during the pressing assessment?

    a. Shoulders elevate
    b. Arms migrate forward
    c. Low back arches
    d. Head migrates forward

11. Which muscle is *most* likely overactive?

    a. Latissimus dorsi
    b. Intrinsic core stabilizers
    c. Gluteus maximus
    d. Middle and lower trapezius

12. Which muscle is *most* likely underactive?

    a. Hip flexors
    b. Erector spinae
    c. Latissimus dorsi
    d. Intrinsic core stabilizers

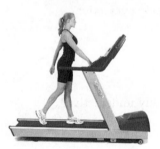

13. What is the *primary* movement compensation demonstrated during the gait assessment?

    a. Shoulders elevate
    b. Feet flatten
    c. Head migrates forward
    d. Low back arches

14. Which muscle is *most* likely overactive?

    a. Erector spinae
    b. Intrinsic core stabilizers
    c. Hamstrings
    d. Gluteus maximus

15. Which muscle is *most* likely underactive?

    a. Hip flexor complex
    b. Latissimus dorsi
    c. Erector spinae
    d. Gluteus maximus

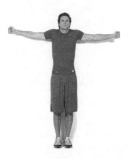

16. What is the *primary* movement compensation demonstrated during the horizontal abduction test?

    a. Shoulders elevate
    b. Elbows flex
    c. Low back arches off wall
    d. Cervical flexion

17. Which muscle is *most* likely overactive?

    a. Rotator cuff
    b. Rhomboids
    c. Middle and lower trapezius
    d. Upper trapezius

18. Which muscle is *most* likely underactive?

    a. Upper trapezius
    b. Levator scapulae
    c. Sternocleidomastoid
    d. Mid and lower trapezius

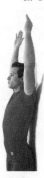

19. What is the *primary* movement compensation demonstrated during the shoulder flexion test?

    a. Shoulders elevate
    b. Elbows flex
    c. Low back arches off wall
    d. Cervical flexion

20. Which muscle is *most* likely overactive?

    a. Rotator cuff
    b. Rhomboids
    c. Middle and lower trapezius
    d. Erector spinae

21. Which muscle is *most* likely underactive?

    a. Erector spinae
    b. Pectoralis major
    c. Rhomboids
    d. Pectoralis minor

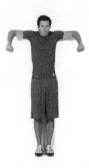

22. What is the *primary* movement compensation demonstrated during the shoulder internal rotation test?

    a. Shoulders elevate
    b. Scapular winging
    c. Low back arches off wall
    d. Cervical retraction

23. Which muscle is *most* likely overactive?

    a. Rotator cuff
    b. Rhomboids
    c. Middle and lower trapezius
    d. Levator scapulae

24. Which muscle is *most* likely underactive?

    a. Upper trapezius
    b. Levator scapulae
    c. Rotator cuff
    d. Pectoralis major

CHAPTER 7

Range of Motion Assessments

EXERCISE 7-1   Essential Vocabulary

PURPOSE: The purpose of this exercise is to have an understanding of key terms used in Chapter 7.

INSTRUCTIONS: Match each term with its proper definition.

VOCABULARY WORDS

1. ___ Range of motion

2. ___ Passive range of motion

3. ___ Active range of motion

DEFINITIONS

A. The amount of motion obtained solely through voluntary contraction from the client.

B. The amount of motion available at a specific joint.

C. The amount of motion obtained by the examiner without any assistance by the client.

EXERCISE 7-2   True/False

INSTRUCTIONS: Choose whether each statement is true or false.

1. Precise neuromuscular control of range of motion at each joint will ultimately decrease excessive stress placed on the body.

   True   False

2. If one joint lacks proper range of motion (ROM), then adjacent joints and tissues (above or below) must move more to compensate for the dysfunctional joint's ROM.

   True   False

3. If an individual possesses less than adequate ankle dorsiflexion, he or she may be at greater risk of injury to the knee, hip, or low back.

   True   False

4. In most normal subjects, active ROM is slightly greater than passive ROM.

   True   False

5. Some joints are constructed so that the joint capsule is the limiting factor in movement whereas other joints rely solely on ligamentous structures for stability.

   True   False

6. A soft end-feel may acknowledge the presence of edema, whereas a firm end-feel may describe increased muscular tonicity.

   True   False

7. Intertester reliability refers to the amount of agreement between goniometric values obtained by the same tester.

   True   False

8. Intratester reliability refers to the amount of agreement between goniometric values obtained by different testers.

   True   False

9. Reliability of joint motion assessment reflects how closely the measurement represents the actual angle or total available range of motion.

   True   False

10. Validity refers to the amount of agreement between successive measurements.

    True   False

EXERCISE 7-3   Matching

INSTRUCTIONS: Identify the different components of a goniometer using the image below.

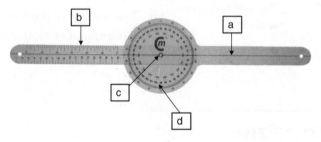

1. ___ Axis
2. ___ Body
3. ___ Stabilization arm
4. ___ Movement arm

EXERCISE 7-4 **Multiple Choice**

INSTRUCTIONS: Answer the questions by referring to the images below.

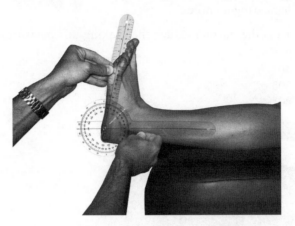

1. What joint motion is being assessed?

   a. Dorsiflexion of the talocrural joint
   b. Plantar flexion of the talocrural joint
   c. Inversion of the talocrural joint
   d. Eversion of the talocrural joint

2. What are the primary muscles being assessed?

   a. Popliteus and sartorius
   b. Gastrocnemius and soleus
   c. Gracilis and biceps femoris
   d. Anterior tibialis and vastus lateralis

3. What is the normal value when taking this measurement?

   a. 0°
   b. 5°
   c. 10°
   d. 20°

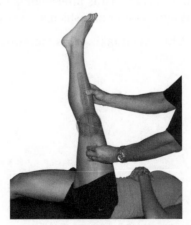

4. What is the primary joint motion being assessed?

   a. Flexion of tibiofemoral joint
   b. Extension of tibiofemoral joint
   c. Abduction of iliofemoral joint
   d. Abduction of tibiofemoral joint

5. All of the following structures are being assessed EXCEPT:

   a. sciatic nerve.
   b. soleus.
   c. gastrocnemius.
   d. hamstring complex.

6. What is the normal value when taking this measurement?

   a. 20°
   b. 40°
   c. 60°
   d. 80°

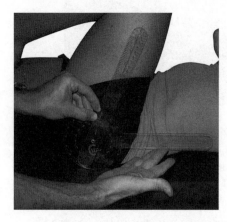

7. What joint motion is being assessed?

   a. Flexion of tibiofemoral joint
   b. Extension of tibiofemoral joint
   c. Flexion of iliofemoral joint
   d. Extension of iliofemoral joint

8. If the client reports a pinching sensation in the front of the hip during this assessment, the

   a. psoas or rectus femoris may be overactive.
   b. gluteus maximus or gluteus medius may be overactive.
   c. vastus medialis oblique and vastus intermedius may be overactive.
   d. semimembranosus and semitendinosus may be overactive.

9. What is the normal value when taking this measurement?

   a. 60°
   b. 80°
   c. 100°
   d. 120°

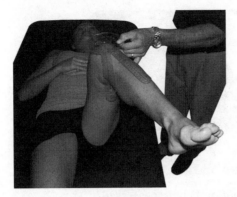

10. What joint motion is being assessed?

    a. Abduction of iliofemoral joint
    b. Adduction of iliofemoral joint
    c. Internal rotation of iliofemoral joint
    d. External rotation of iliofemoral joint

11. All of the following muscles and ligaments are being assessed EXCEPT:

    a. piriformis and hip external rotators.
    b. adductor magnus (oblique fibers) and ischiofemoral ligament.
    c. gluteus medius (posterior fibers) and gluteus maximus.
    d. adductor complex and medial hamstring complex.

12. What is the normal value when taking this measurement?

    a. 25°
    b. 45°
    c. 65°
    d. 85°

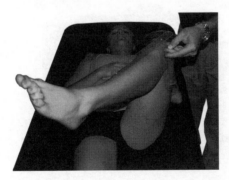

13. What joint motion is being assessed?

    a. Abduction of iliofemoral joint
    b. Adduction of iliofemoral joint
    c. Internal rotation of iliofemoral joint
    d. External rotation of iliofemoral joint

14. What antagonists are potentially underactive if range of motion is limited?

    a. Piriformis, hip external rotators, and adductor magnus (oblique fibers)
    b. Tensor fascia latae, rectus femoris, and psoas major
    c. Adductor longus, adductor brevis, and adductor magnus (anterior fibers)
    d. Pectineus, gracilis, and gluteus medius (anterior fibers)

15. What is the normal value when taking this measurement?

    a. 25°
    b. 45°
    c. 65°
    d. 85°

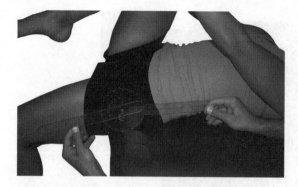

16. What joint motion is being assessed?

    a. Flexion of iliofemoral joint
    b. Extension of iliofemoral joint
    c. Internal rotation of iliofemoral joint
    d. External rotation of iliofemoral joint

17. All of the following muscles and tissues are being assessed EXCEPT:

    a. psoas, iliacus, and rectus femoris.
    b. tensor fascia latae and sartorius.
    c. adductor complex and anterior hip capsule.
    d. gluteus minimus, biceps femoris (short head), and semimembranosus.

18. What is the normal value when taking this measurement?

    a. 0° to –10°
    b. 5°
    c. 10°
    d. 20°

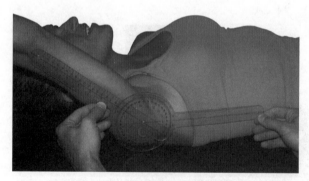

19. What joint motion is being assessed?

    a. Flexion of shoulder complex
    b. Extension of shoulder complex
    c. Internal rotation of shoulder complex
    d. External rotation of shoulder complex

20. What are the primary muscles being assessed?

    a. Biceps brachii, anterior deltoid, and middle deltoid
    b. Latissimus dorsi, teres major, and teres minor
    c. Pectoralis major (upper fibers and clavicular fibers)
    d. Lower trapezius, middle trapezius, and rhomboids

21. What is the normal value when taking this measurement?

    a. 0°
    b. 60°
    c. 100°
    d. 160°

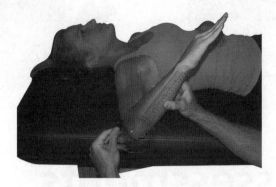

22. What joint motion is being assessed?

    a. Flexion of glenohumeral joint
    b. Extension of glenohumeral joint
    c. Internal rotation of glenohumeral joint
    d. External rotation of glenohumeral joint

23. Which muscles and structures are being assessed?

    a. Infraspinatus, teres minor, and posterior glenohumeral joint capsule
    b. Rhomboids, levator scapulae, and scalenes
    c. Pectoralis major (lower fibers) and triceps (long head)
    d. Latissimus dorsi, medial deltoid, and pectoralis minor

24. What is the normal value when taking this measurement?

    a. 15°
    b. 30°
    c. 45°
    d. 60°

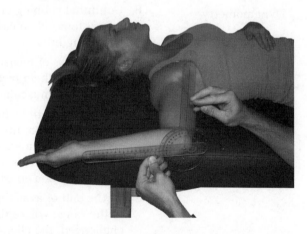

25. What joint motion is being assessed?

    a. Flexion of glenohumeral joint
    b. Extension of glenohumeral joint
    c. Internal rotation of glenohumeral joint
    d. External rotation of glenohumeral joint

26. What is the normal value when taking this measurement?

    a. 30°
    b. 60°
    c. 90°
    d. 120°

CHAPTER 8

Strength Assessments

EXERCISE 8-1 **Essential Vocabulary**

PURPOSE: The purpose of this exercise is to have an understanding of key terms used in Chapter 8.

INSTRUCTIONS: Match each term with its proper definition.

VOCABULARY WORDS

1. ___ Strength

2. ___ Isokinetic testing

3. ___ Dynamometry

4. ___ IT band syndrome

5. ___ Break test

DEFINITIONS

A. The ability of the neuromuscular system to produce internal tension to overcome an external force.

B. Continual rubbing of the IT band over the lateral femoral epicondyle leading to the area becoming inflamed.

C. The process of measuring forces at work using a handheld instrument that measures the force of muscular contraction.

D. Muscle strength testing performed with a specialized apparatus that provides variable resistance to a movement, so that no matter how much effort is exerted, the movement takes place at a constant speed.

E. At the end of available range, or at a point in the range where the muscle is most challenged, the client is asked to hold that position and not allow the examiner to break the hold with manual resistance.

EXERCISE 8-2 **True/False**

INSTRUCTIONS: Choose whether each statement is true or false.

1. The ability of the nervous system to recruit and activate muscles dictates muscle strength.
   True **False**

2. One must be a qualified health and fitness professional (i.e., licensed professional) to apply manual muscle testing techniques on clients.

   True   False

3. Manual muscle testing is more objective and reliable than isokinetic testing and handheld dynamometry.

   True   False

4. Manual muscle testing provides an opportunity to assess muscle function with low cost and difficulty.

   True   False

5. Overactivity of a shortened muscle will reciprocally inhibit its functional antagonist leading to a false reading that a muscle is weak when in fact the strength impression is purely a factor of joint position.

   True   False

6. Manual muscle testing is an assessment process used to test the recruitment capacity and contraction quality of individual muscles or movements.

   True   False

7. In addition to tight muscles, restrictions in skin, neural tissue, and articular ligaments can also result in muscle inhibition.

   True   False

8. The numeric grade of 1 represents a client who maintains good structural alignment and holds the end-range position against the assessor's pressure.

   True   False

9. A numeric grade of 3 indicates little to no ability of the client to withstand or resist pressure from the assessor.

   True   False

10. Muscle weakness can be related to several factors, but the most common factors in a healthy individual are atrophy and inhibition.

    True   False

EXERCISE 8-3   Multiple Choice

INSTRUCTIONS: Answer the questions below. For questions 3 through 20, answer the questions by referring to the images.

1. Step 1 of the NASM manual muscle testing process includes all of the following EXCEPT:
   a. place the joint in the desired position and ask the client to hold that position while applying pressure against the limb directly in the line of pull for the desired muscle.
   b. the pressure applied should be done in a ramping-up manner versus quickly applying maximal force.
   c. the client must hold that position for four seconds and not allow the assessor to "break" the hold.
   d. place the muscle in a maximally lengthened position and retest.

2. To improve reliability and safety, as well as reduce errors with a manual muscle test, the following guidelines should be followed EXCEPT:

    a. the same health and fitness professional should be used with a single client to reduce intertester variability.
    b. manual resistance should be applied at a 45-degree angle to the primary axis of a body part.
    c. not testing a muscle in a fully lengthened position because it can lead to overstretching and injury.
    d. establishing a time (four seconds) for the client to hold the isometric muscle contraction.

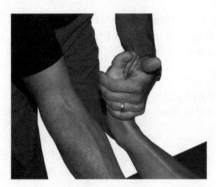

3. What is the prime mover being assessed?

    a. Anterior tibialis
    b. Posterior tibialis
    c. Soleus
    d. Gastrocnemius

4. To execute the test, the health and fitness professional should apply gradual and increasing pressure to the medial dorsal surface of the foot in the direction of

    a. plantarflexion and eversion.
    b. dorsiflexion and inversion.
    c. dorsiflexion and eversion.
    d. plantarflexion and inversion.

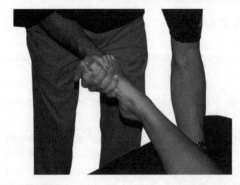

5. What is the prime mover being assessed?

    a. Anterior tibialis
    b. Posterior tibialis
    c. Soleus
    d. Gastrocnemius

6. To execute the test, the health and fitness professional should apply gradual and increasing pressure to the medial plantar surface of the foot in the direction of

   a. plantarflexion and eversion.
   b. dorsiflexion and inversion.
   c. dorsiflexion and eversion.
   d. plantarflexion and inversion.

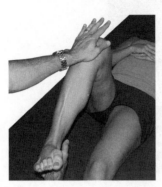

7. What are the prime movers being assessed?

   a. Semimembranosus and semitendinosus
   b. Anterior tibialis and posterior tibialis
   c. Rectus femoris and vastus lateralis
   d. Gastrocnemius and soleus

8. What are potentially overactive muscles if strength is limited?

   a. Semimembranosus and semitendinosus
   b. Anterior tibialis and posterior tibialis
   c. Quadriceps and biceps femoris
   d. Popliteus and gracilis

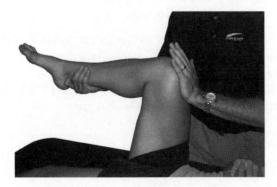

9. What are the prime movers being assessed?

   a. Medial hamstring complex
   b. Iliacus and psoas major
   c. Gluteus maximus and sartorius
   d. Popliteus and gracilis

10. To execute the test, the health and fitness professional should apply gradual and increasing pressure at the distal end of the femur in the direction of
    a. hip extension.
    b. hip flexion
    c. hip adduction.
    d. hip abduction.

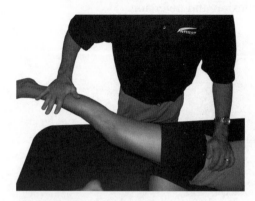

11. What is the prime mover being assessed?
    a. Semitendinosus
    b. Psoas major
    c. Gracilis
    d. Gluteus medius

12. To execute the test, the health and fitness professional should apply gradual and increasing pressure to the lateral aspect of the lower leg just above the ankle joint in the direction of
    a. hip flexion and adduction.
    b. hip flexion and abduction.
    c. hip extension and adduction.
    d. hip extension and abduction.

13. What are some potentially overactive muscles if strength is limited?
    a. Semimembranosus and semitendinosus
    b. Anterior tibialis and posterior tibialis
    c. Adductor complex and hip flexor complex (TFL, iliopsoas, rectus femoris)
    d. Popliteus and vastus medialis oblique

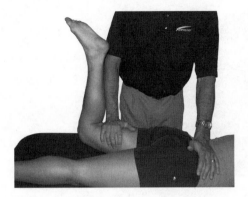

14. What is the prime mover being assessed?

    a. Pectineus
    b. Psoas major
    c. Gluteus maximus
    d. Gracilis

15. To execute the test, the health and fitness professional should apply gradual and increasing pressure to the upper leg just above the knee in the direction of

    a. hip flexion, adduction, and internal rotation.
    b. hip flexion, abduction, and external rotation.
    c. hip extension, adduction, and internal rotation.
    d. hip extension, abduction, and external rotation.

16. What are some potentially overactive muscles if strength is limited?

    a. Medial gastrocnemius and gluteus medius (anterior fibers)
    b. Anterior tibialis and posterior tibialis
    c. Iliopsoas, rectus femoris, adductor longus/brevis, and pectineus
    d. Popliteus, gracilis, and semitendinosus

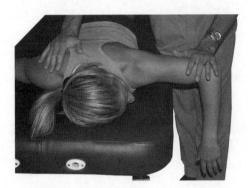

17. What is the prime mover being assessed?

    a. Pectoralis major
    b. Rhomboids
    c. Pectoralis minor
    d. Triceps brachii

18. To execute the test, the health and fitness professional should apply gradual and increasing pressure to the distal humerus just above the elbow in a

    a. downward direction toward the floor.
    b. upward direction toward the ceiling.
    c. shoulder extension and internal rotation.
    d. shoulder flexion and external rotation.

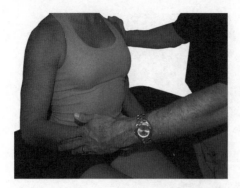

19. What are the prime movers being assessed?

    a. Shoulder external rotators (infraspinatus and teres minor)
    b. Rhomboids and lower trapezius
    c. Pectoralis minor and serratus anterior
    d. Anterior deltoid and pectoralis major

20. To execute the test, the health and fitness professional should apply gradual and increasing pressure to the lower arm just above the wrist in the direction of

    a. shoulder external rotation.
    b. shoulder flexion.
    c. shoulder extension.
    d. shoulder internal rotation.

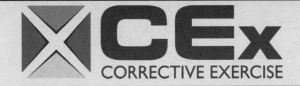

THE CORRECTIVE EXERCISE CONTINUUM

CHAPTER 9

Inhibitory Techniques

EXERCISE 9-1   Essential Vocabulary

PURPOSE: The purpose of this exercise is to have an understanding of key terms used in Chapter 9.

INSTRUCTIONS: Match each term with its proper definition.

VOCABULARY WORDS

1. ___ Self-myofascial release
2. ___ Davis's law
3. ___ Relative flexibility
4. ___ Autogenic inhibition
5. ___ Gamma loop

DEFINITIONS

A. Soft tissue will model along the lines of stress.

B. A flexibility technique used to inhibit over-active muscle fibers.

C. The reflex arc consisting of small anterior horn nerve cells and their small fibers that project to the intrafusal bundle to produce its contraction, which initiates the afferent impulses that pass through the posterior root to the anterior horn cells, inducing, in turn, reflex contraction of the entire muscle.

D. Inhibition of the muscle spindle resulting from the Golgi tendon organ stimulation.

E. The phenomenon of the human movement system seeking the path of least resistance during functional movement patterns (or movement compensation).

EXERCISE 9-2   True/False

INSTRUCTIONS: Choose whether each statement is true or false.

1. Evidence supporting the rationale for using self-myofascial release (SMR) for flexibility purposes is derived from research on ischemic compression and myofascial release techniques.

    True   False

2. Any trauma to the tissue of the body creates inflammation. Inflammation in turn activates the body's pain receptors and initiates a protective mechanism, increasing muscle tension or causing muscle spasm.

   True   False

3. Adhesions (i.e., knots or trigger points) can begin to form permanent structural changes in the soft tissue that is evidenced by Davis's law.

   True   False

4. Self-myofascial release techniques may help in releasing the microspasms that develop in traumatized tissue and break up the facial adhesions that are created through the cumulative injury cycle process.

   True   False

5. Self-myofascial release is believed to stimulate receptors located throughout the muscle, fascia, and connective tissues (Golgi tendon organ, interstitial receptors, and Ruffini endings) through sustained pressure to produce an inhibitory response to the muscle spindle and decrease gamma loop activity.

   True   False

6. Type III and type IV receptors (interstitial receptors) in conjunction with Ruffini endings have been shown to have autonomic functions that include changes in heart rate, blood pressure, respiration, and tissue viscosity.

   True   False

7. Decreasing vasodilation improves the ability of tissues to receive adequate amounts of oxygen and nutrients as well as removal of waste byproducts (via the bloodstream) to facilitate tissue recovery and repair.

   True   False

8. Faulty breathing patterns (shallow chest breathing) can lead to synergistic dominance of secondary breathing muscles.

   True   False

9. The autonomic nervous system's response to sustained pressure increases global muscle tonus as well as fluid dynamics to increase viscosity and the tonus of the smooth muscle cells located in fascia.

   True   False

10. Increasing sympathetic tone reduces the prolonged faulty contraction of muscle tissue that can lead to the cumulative injury cycle.

    True   False

11. Individuals who have never performed self-myofascial release should begin by using a dense and rigid roller (such as a PVC roller) because it offers increased penetration into the soft tissue.

    True   False

12. Progression when using balls as a self-myofascial release tool should be made by beginning with a large diameter ball (i.e., medicine ball), then going to a smaller diameter, firmer ball (i.e., tennis ball, softball, baseball, golf ball).

    True   False

13. At the current time, there are no known reasons that self-myofascial release cannot be performed on a daily basis.

    True   False

14. Individuals performing self-myofascial release should hold the foam roller on a tender area for roughly 30 seconds at high intensity (maximal pain tolerance) and 90 seconds for lower intensity (minimum pain tolerance) before moving to the next region.

True **False**

15. Precautionary measures do not apply for self-myofascial release techniques, and it is considered safe for all populations including people with organ failure, bleeding disorders, cancer, and contagious skin conditions.

True **False**

EXERCISE 9-3 | **Multiple Choice**

INSTRUCTIONS: Review the image, then answer the following questions.

1. What is the *primary* muscle being addressed in the image below?

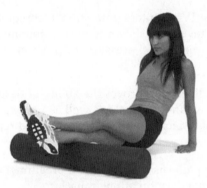

    a. Biceps femoris
    b. Rectus femoris
    c. Gastrocnemius
    d. Anterior tibialis

2. What is the *primary* muscle being addressed in the image below?

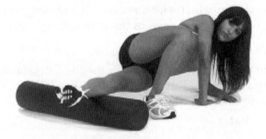

    a. Peroneals
    b. Tensor fascia latae
    c. Popliteus
    d. Anterior tibialis

3. What is the *primary* region being addressed in the image below?

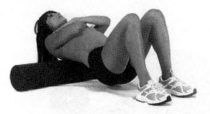

   a. Thoracic spine
   b. Lumbar spine
   c. Cervical spine
   d. Serratus anterior

4. What is the *primary* muscle being addressed in the image below?

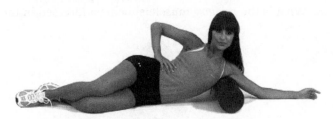

   a. Pectoralis minor
   b. Latissimus dorsi
   c. Pectoralis major
   d. Anterior deltoid

5. What is the *primary* muscle being addressed in the image below?

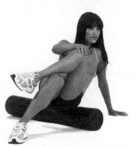

   a. Tensor fascia latae
   b. Psoas
   c. Piriformis
   d. Rectus femoris

6. What is the *primary* muscle(s) being addressed in the image below?

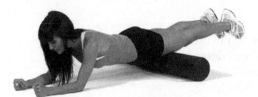

   a. IT-band
   b. Quadriceps
   c. Peroneals
   d. Adductors

7. What is the *primary* muscle(s) being addressed in the image below?

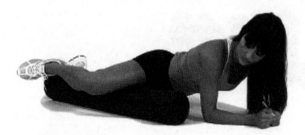

    a. Adductors
    b. Rectus femoris
    c. IT-band
    d. Tensor fascia latae

8. What is the *primary* muscle(s) being addressed in the image below?

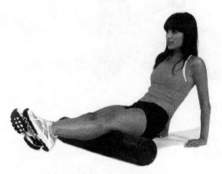

    a. Hamstring complex
    b. Rectus femoris
    c. IT-band
    d. Tensor fascia latae

9. What is the *primary* muscle being addressed in the image below?

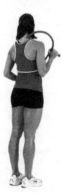

    a. Upper Trapezius
    b. Latissimus dorsi
    c. Sternocleidomastoid
    d. Coracobrachialis

10. What is the *primary* region being addressed in the image below?

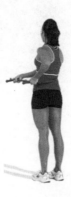

a. Thoracic spine
b. Lumbar spine
c. Cervical spine
d. Sacrum

EXERCISE 9-4   # Fill in the Blank

INSTRUCTIONS: Fill in the empty spaces in the chart below.

ACUTE VARIABLES FOR SELF-MYOFASCIAL RELEASE			
Frequency	Sets	Repetitions	Duration
	1	N/A	

CHAPTER 10

Lengthening Techniques

EXERCISE 10-1   Essential Vocabulary

PURPOSE: The purpose of this exercise is to have an understanding of key terms used in Chapter 10.

INSTRUCTIONS: Match each term with its proper definition.

VOCABULARY WORDS

1. ___ Autogenic inhibition

2. ___ Recurrent inhibition

3. ___ Stretch reflex

DEFINITIONS

A. The process when neural impulses that sense tension are greater than the impulses that cause muscles to contract, providing an inhibitory effect to the muscle spindles.

B. A muscle contraction in response to stretching within the muscle.

C. A feedback circuit that can decrease the excitability of motor neurons via the interneuron called the Renshaw cell.

EXERCISE 10-2   True/False

INSTRUCTIONS: Choose whether each statement is true or false.

1. The second phase in the corrective exercise continuum is to lengthen overactive or tight neuromyofascial tissues.

   True   False

2. Although the exact mechanisms responsible for the efficacy of static stretching are not fully understood, it is believed that static stretching may produce both mechanical and neural adaptations that result in increased range of motion.

   True   False

3. The ability of an individual to perform static stretching without assistance and the slow-minimal to no motion required has led this form of flexibility training to be associated with the lowest risk for injury during the stretching routine and deemed the safest to use.

   True   False

4. Neurologically, static stretching of neuromyofascial tissue to the end range of motion appears to decrease motor neuron excitability, possibly through the inhibitory effects from the Golgi tendon organs (autogenic inhibition) as well as possible contribution from the Renshaw recurrent loop (recurrent inhibition).

   True   False

5. Mechanically, static stretching appears to affect the viscoelastic component of neuromyofascial tissue, decreasing the passive resistance a muscle has to a stretch force throughout most of the range of motion.

   True   False

6. In general, it is thought that static stretching for 5 to 10 seconds causes an acute viscoelastic stress relaxation response, allowing for an immediate increase in range of motion.

   True   False

7. Increasing musculotendinous flexibility through stretching will lead to a decrease muscle energy absorption and trauma to muscle fibers with a decrease in injury risk being the potential result.

   True   False

8. Decreasing muscle stiffness through stretching will decrease the work required to perform a particular activity and potentially increase overall performance.

   True   False

9. Stretching exercises are primarily used to increase the available range of motion (ROM) at a particular joint, specifically if the ROM at that joint is limited by tight neuromyofascial tissues.

   True   False

10. The scientific literature does not support the use of stretching exercises to achieve increased joint range of motion.

    True   False

11. Several researchers suggest that each joint and muscle group may respond similarly to stretching protocols; thus stretching protocols may not need to be different for each range of motion (ROM) limitation found.

    True   False

12. A tight or shortened hip flexor group may create an anterior pelvic tilt, causing the hamstring complex to be lengthened under normal resting positions, which may inhibit normal hip flexion range of motion.

    True   False

13. Reviews of the best available research suggest that, acutely, stretching may have a detrimental effect on muscular strength and power.

    True   False

14. The current evidence suggests that acute pre-exercise stretching has a significant impact on injury risk although the effects of chronic, long-term stretching protocols tend to lead to increased injury rates.
    True   False

15. Recent research suggests that range of motion (ROM) can be improved via the application of heat or ice (either heating or cooling the tissue), suggesting that warming-up of tissues is not necessary to improve ROM.
    True   False

16. There is moderate evidence to indicate that regular stretching improves range of motion, strength, and performance, and decreases injury risk in healthy individuals without identified limitations in flexibility.
    True   False

17. There is moderate evidence to indicate that acute, pre-exercise stretching performed in isolation decreases strength and performance and does not affect injury risk in healthy individuals without identified limitations in flexibility.
    True   False

18. Studies have found that stretching reduces both physiologic (electromyographic) and self-reported muscle tension, results in a decreased feeling of sadness, and can decrease the levels of stress-related hormones.
    True   False

19. Contraindications for applying stretching techniques include osteoporosis, acute rheumatoid arthritis, and acute injury or muscle strain or tear.
    True   False

20. In a corrective exercise program, static stretching should only be applied to muscles that have been determined to be underactive, weak, or lengthened during the assessment process.
    True   False

PURPOSE: To understand neuromuscular stretching as discussed in Chapter 10.

21. Most of the current research has demonstrated that neuromuscular stretching is not as effective at increasing range of motion when compared with static stretching.
    True   False

22. Neuromuscular stretching is a technique that involves a process of isometrically contracting a desired muscle in a lengthened position to induce a relaxation response on the tissue, allowing it to further elongate.
    True   False

23. It is believed that the isometric contraction used during neuromuscular stretching increases motor neuron excitability as a result of stimulation to the muscle spindle and that this leads to an increased resistance to a change in length (or, ability to increase length of tissue).
    True   False

24. The premise behind neuromuscular stretching (NMS) is very similar to static stretching; however, NMS usually requires the assistance of another person, and thus it is traditionally used under the supervision of a health and fitness professional.

    True   **False**

25. Neuromuscular stretching can be performed daily unless otherwise stated.

    True   **False**

26. Neuromuscular stretching is commonly called proprioceptive neuromuscular facilitation (PNF).

    True   **False**

27. Neuromuscular stretching involves taking the muscle to its end range of motion (ROM), actively contracting the muscle to be stretched for 5 to 10 seconds, then passively moving the joint to a new end ROM and holding this position for 20 to 30 seconds.

    True   **False**

28. Typically neuromuscular stretching involves the aid of a partner to provide a resistance to the active muscle contraction and passively stretch the joint into the new range of motion.

    True   **False**

29. Acute static stretching held for at least 30 seconds does appear to decrease muscular strength and power, whereas ballistic or neuromuscular stretching does not have the same effect.

    True   **False**

30. Like static stretching, neuromuscular stretching should only be applied to muscles that have been determined to be overactive or tight during the assessment.

    True   **False**

EXERCISE 10-3   **Multiple Choice**

INSTRUCTIONS: Review the image then answer the following questions.

1. What is the *primary* muscle being stretched in the image below?

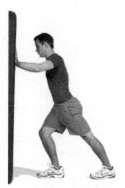

   a. Biceps femoris
   b. Rectus femoris
   c. Gastrocnemius
   d. Anterior tibialis

2. What is the *primary* muscle being stretched in the image below?

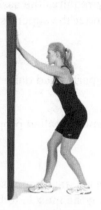

    a. Soleus
    b. Tensor fascia latae
    c. Posterior tibialis
    d. Anterior tibialis

3. What is the *primary* muscle being stretched in the image below?

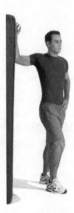

    a. Pectoralis major
    b. Rhomboids
    c. Posterior deltoid
    d. Supraspinatus

4. What is the *primary* muscle being stretched in the image below?

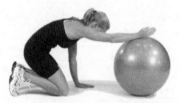

    a. Pectoralis minor
    b. Latissimus dorsi
    c. Pectoralis major
    d. Anterior deltoid

5. What is the *primary* muscle being stretched in the image below?

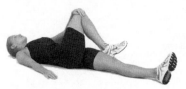

    a. Tensor fascia latae
    b. Psoas
    c. Piriformis
    d. Rectus femoris

6. What is the *primary* muscle being stretched in the image below?

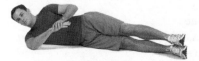

    a. Pectoralis major
    b. Posterior deltoid
    c. Erector spinae
    d. Anterior deltoid

7. What is the *primary* muscle being stretched in the image below?

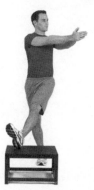

    a. Biceps femoris
    b. Rectus femoris
    c. Adductor magnus
    d. Tensor fascia latae

8. What is the *primary* muscle being stretched in the image below?

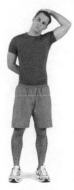

    a. Levator scapulae
    b. Sternocleidomastoid
    c. Upper trapezius
    d. Pectoralis minor

9. What is the *primary* muscle being stretched in the image below?

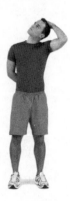

    a. Levator scapulae
    b. Sternocleidomastoid
    c. Upper trapezius
    d. Pectoralis minor

10. What is the *primary* muscle being stretched in the image below?

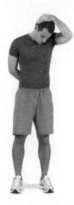

    a. Levator scapulae
    b. Sternocleidomastoid
    c. Upper trapezius
    d. Rectus capitis

PURPOSE: To understand neuromuscular stretching as discussed in Chapter 10.

11. What neuromuscular stretch (NMS) is being demonstrated in the image below?

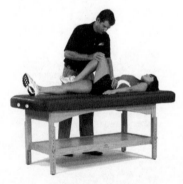

    a. NMS gastrocnemius/soleus complex
    b. NMS hip flexor complex
    c. NMS hamstring complex
    d. NMS piriformis

12. What neuromuscular stretch (NMS) is being demonstrated in the image below?

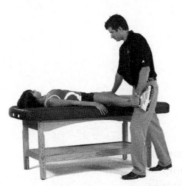

    a. NMS adductor complex (straight knee)
    b. NMS hip flexor complex
    c. NMS hamstring complex
    d. NMS piriformis

13. What neuromuscular stretch (NMS) is being demonstrated in the image below?

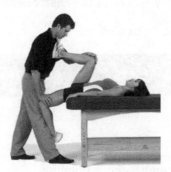

    a. NMS adductor complex (straight knee)
    b. NMS hip flexor complex
    c. NMS hamstring complex
    d. NMS piriformis

14. What neuromuscular stretch (NMS) is being demonstrated in the image below?

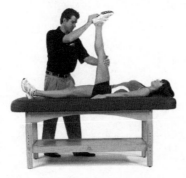

    a. NMS adductor complex (straight knee)
    b. NMS hip flexor complex
    c. NMS hamstring complex
    d. NMS gastrocnemius/soleus complex

15. What neuromuscular stretch (NMS) is being demonstrated in the image below?

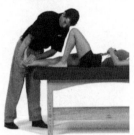

    a. NMS adductor complex (straight knee)
    b. NMS hip flexor complex
    c. NMS hamstring complex
    d. NMS gastrocnemius/soleus complex

EXERCISE 10-4   Practical Application

INSTRUCTIONS: Fill in the empty spaces in the charts below.

A. Acute Variables for Static Stretching

FREQUENCY (PER WEEK)	SETS	REPETITIONS	DURATION OF EACH REPETITION
Daily (unless specified otherwise)	N/A		

B. Acute Variables for Neuromuscular Stretching

FREQUENCY (PER WEEK)	SETS	REPETITIONS	DURATION OF EACH REPETITION
	N/A	1–3	

CHAPTER 11

Activation and Integration Techniques

EXERCISE 11-1   Essential Vocabulary

PURPOSE: The purpose of this exercise is to have an understanding of key terms used in Chapter 11.

INSTRUCTIONS: Match each term with its proper definition.

VOCABULARY WORDS

1. ___ Intramuscular coordination

2. ___ Motor unit activation

3. ___ Synchronization

4. ___ Firing rate

5. ___ Intermuscular coordination

DEFINITIONS

A. The ability of the neuromuscular system to allow optimal levels of motor unit recruitment and synchronization within a muscle.

B. The synergistic activation of multiple motor units.

C. The ability of the neuromuscular system to allow all muscles to work together with proper activation and timing between them.

D. The progressive activation of a muscle by successive recruitment of contractile units (motor units) to accomplish increasing gradations of contractile strength.

E. The frequency at which a motor unit is activated.

EXERCISE 11-2   True/False

INSTRUCTIONS: Choose whether each statement is true or false.

1. Activation refers to the stimulation (or reeducation) of underactive myofascial tissue.

   True   **False**

2. The use of multiple joint actions and multiple muscle synergies helps to reestablish neuromuscular control, promoting coordinated movement among the involved muscles.

True   False

3. Isolated strengthening is a technique used to increase intermuscular coordination of specific muscle groups.

True   False

4. The eccentric component involved with isolated strengthening has been proven to play a role in the recovery of muscle injury and tendinopathies, and in preparation for integrated training.

True   False

5. Integrated dynamic movement enhances the functional capacity of the human movement system by increasing multiplanar neuromuscular control.

True   False

6. Multi-joint motions versus single-joint motions promote and require greater intermuscular coordination.

True   False

7. Research has shown that the short-term use of unilateral exercises is ineffective at increasing performance measures.

True   False

8. Overhead movements, often used in integrated dynamic movements, help to place increased stress on the core musculature.

True   False

9. Resistance training performed on unstable surfaces may be challenging and should not be considered as an effective mode to improve a client's movement patterns.

True   False

10. Integrated dynamic movement performed within a corrective exercise program should involve heavy loads with an explosive tempo to maximize postural stabilization.

True   False

EXERCISE 11-3   Multiple Choice

INSTRUCTIONS: Select the best answer from the choices given for each question.

1. All of the following are reasons to perform inhibitory and lengthening techniques before isolated strengthening EXCEPT:

   a. When a joint is not free to move, the muscles that move it cannot be free to move it.

   b. Muscles can be restored to normal even if the joints that they move are not free to move.

   c. Normal muscle function is dependent on normal joint movement.

   d. Impaired muscle function perpetuates and may cause deterioration in abnormal joints.

2. What is the MOST appropriate repetition tempo during isolated strengthening exercises?

   a. 1 second isometric hold at end-range and 1 second eccentric action
   b. 2 seconds isometric hold at end-range and 2 seconds eccentric action
   c. 2 seconds isometric hold at end-range and 4 seconds eccentric action
   d. 4 seconds isometric hold at end-range and 4 seconds eccentric action

3. Isolated strengthening exercises are used to isolate particular muscles to increase the force production capabilities through

   a. concentric and eccentric muscle actions.
   b. isometric muscle actions.
   c. isotonic muscle actions.
   d. isokinetic muscle actions.

4. Isolated strengthening is a technique used to increase intramuscular coordination of specific muscles through a combination of all of the following EXCEPT:

   a. enhanced motor unit activation.
   b. enhanced motor unit synchronization.
   c. enhanced motor unit firing rate.
   d. enhanced relative flexibility.

5. Which of the following is an example of an isolated strengthening exercise for the hip?

   a. Wall slides
   b. Prone iso-abs
   c. Floor cobra
   d. Ball combo 2 with dowel rod

6. Which of the following is an example of an isolated strengthening exercise for the intrinsic core stabilizers?

   a. Towel scrunches
   b. Chin tucks with blood pressure cuff
   c. Squat to row
   d. Side iso-abs

7. Which of the following is an example of an isolated strengthening exercise for the shoulder?

   a. Single-arm row to arrow position
   b. Quadruped arm/opposite leg raise
   c. Standing cable external rotation
   d. Ball squat to overhead press

8. It is suggested that many injuries occur during _____ in the frontal and transverse planes.

   a. concentric acceleration
   b. eccentric deceleration
   c. eccentric acceleration
   d. concentric deceleration

9. Multi-joint motions promote and require greater

   a. intermuscular coordination.
   b. relative flexibility.
   c. synergistic dominance.
   d. autogenic inhibition.

10. Which of the following is an appropriate progression when using integrated dynamic movement?

    a. Ball wall squat → step-up → lunge → single-leg squat
    b. Step-up → ball wall squat → lunge → single-leg squat
    c. Lunge → step-up → ball wall squat → single-leg squat
    d. Ball wall squat → single-leg squat → lunge→ step-up

INSTRUCTIONS: Choose the letter that correctly answers these questions about positional isometrics.

11. The purpose of positional isometrics is to increase the _____ of specific muscles necessary to heighten activation levels before integrating them back into their functional synergies.

    a. intermuscular coordination
    b. intramuscular coordination
    c. autogenic inhibition
    d. reciprocal inhibition

12. Positional isometrics can be used as needed and consists of _____ set of _____ repetitions.

    a. one, two
    b. one, four
    c. two, six
    d. two, eight

13. Positional isometrics are used to heighten the activation of _____ muscle(s) of a joint.

    a. underactive
    b. overactive
    c. hypertonic
    d. tight

14. Isometric muscle contractions generate _____ levels of tension than concentric muscle contractions and provide functional strength at approximately _____ degrees on either side of the joint angle of contraction.

    a. higher, 10
    b. lower, 20
    c. equal, 50
    d. lower, 70

15. What is the proper sequence of intensity when performing positional isometrics?

    a. 25% → 50% → 75% → 100%
    b. 20% → 40% → 60% → 80%
    c. 15% → 30% → 45% → 60%
    d. 10% → 20% → 30% → 40%

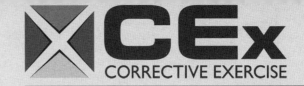

CORRECTIVE EXERCISE STRATEGIES

CHAPTER 12

Corrective Strategies for Foot and Ankle Impairments

EXERCISE 12-1   Essential Vocabulary

PURPOSE: The purpose of this exercise is to have an understanding of key terms used in Chapter 12.

INSTRUCTIONS: Match each term with its proper definition.

VOCABULARY WORDS

1. ___ Plantar fasciitis

2. ___ Tendinopathy

3. ___ Tendinosis

4. ___ Periosteum

5. ___ Ankle sprain

6. ___ Medial tibial stress syndrome

7. ___ Chronic ankle instability

8. ___ Pes planus

9. ___ Pes cavus

DEFINITIONS

A. A combination of pain, swelling, and impaired performance commonly associated with the Achilles' tendon.

B. Pain in the front of the tibia caused by an overload to the tibia and the associated musculature.

C. A membrane that lines the outer surface of all bones.

D. Irritation and swelling of the thick tissue on the bottom of the foot. The most common complaint is pain in the bottom of the heel.

E. Damage to a tendon at a cellular level, but does not present to inflammation.

F. An injury to the ankle ligaments in which small tears occur in the ligaments.

G. A flattened medial arch during weight-bearing.

H. Repetitive episodes of giving way at the ankle, coupled with feelings of instability.

I. A high medial arch when weight-bearing.

▌EXERCISE 12-2   **True/False**

INSTRUCTIONS: Choose whether each statement is true or false.

1. Compensation or dysfunction in one region, such as the foot and ankle, may lead to dysfunctions in other areas of the body.

    True   False

2. The foot and ankle complex must withstand a high amount of contact force (ground reaction force) with each step taken as it is closest to the impact site (foot strike).

    True   False

3. The tarsal bones consist of the cuboid, medial, intermediate, and lateral cuneiforms, navicular, talus, and calcaneus.

    True   False

4. The subtalar joint consists of the talus and tibia.

    True   False

5. The talocrural joint (tibia, fibula, and talus) is commonly called the ankle joint.

    True   False

6. The transverse arch consists of the cuboid and cuneiforms.

    True   False

7. The medial longitudinal arch is made up of the proximal, middle, and distal phalanges.

    True   False

8. Lack of ankle dorsiflexion, an increased body mass index, and a pronated foot type have been associated with plantar fasciitis.

    True   False

9. The plantar fascia is a thick, fibrous band of tissue that runs from the calcaneus and fans out to insert on the metatarsal heads to support the longitudinal arch of the foot.

    True   False

10. The gastrocnemius complex, which consists of the gastrocnemius and soleus muscles, share a common Achilles' tendon that inserts on the base of the talus.

    True   False

▌EXERCISE 12-3   **Multiple Choice**

INSTRUCTIONS: Select the best answer from the choices given for each question.

1. All of the following are risk factors for medial tibial stress syndrome EXCEPT:

    a. excessive running or training.
    b. lack of muscular endurance of the calf musculature.
    c. overpronation of the foot/ankle.
    d. 20° of ankle dorsiflexion.

2. Lateral ankle sprains are the most common type of sprain, and PRIMARILY affect the lateral ankle ligaments, including the

   a. anterior talofibular ligament, calcaneofibular ligament, and posterior talofibular ligament.
   b. lateral collateral ligament, medial collateral ligament, and anterior cruciate ligament.
   c. dorsal tarsometatarsal ligament, dorsal cuneonavicular ligament, and dorsal talonavicular ligament.
   d. medial talocalcaneal ligament, plantar calcaneonavicular ligament, and posterior talocalcaneal ligament.

3. Risk factors for ankle sprain include all of the following EXCEPT:

   a. decreased ankle dorsiflexion range of motion.
   b. previous ankle sprain.
   c. women with increased calcaneal eversion range of motion.
   d. stretching the calf musculature before activity.

4. Musculature imbalance and tightness of the lower leg is theorized to contribute to knee valgus, specifically tightness of the lateral ankle musculature including the

   a. lateral gastrocnemius, soleus, and peroneals.
   b. medial gastrocnemius, anterior tibialis, and posterior tibialis.
   c. gracilis, popliteus, and semimembranosus.
   d. sartorius, semitendinosus, and flexor digitorum longus.

5. Pes planus (increased pronation) is characterized by all of the following EXCEPT:

   a. flattening, externally rotating, and everting of the feet.
   b. knee valgus.
   c. internal rotation of the femur.
   d. a high medial arch during weight-bearing activities.

6. If the knees come together during the squat (medial knee displacement) the individual may have all of the following EXCEPT:

   a. decreased calf flexibility.
   b. greater hip external range of motion.
   c. increased hip abductor strength.
   d. decreased plantar flexion strength.

7. According to the text, key goniometric assessments to determine range of motion deficiencies that may be contributing to foot and ankle dysfunction include all of the following EXCEPT:

   a. first metatarsophalangeal joint.
   b. ankle dorsiflexion.
   c. hip extension.
   d. glenohumeral internal rotation.

8. Key regions to inhibit via foam rolling for an individual with a foot/ankle impairment(s) include the

   a. soleus/lateral gastrocnemius, peroneals, biceps femoris, and tensor fascia latae.
   b. medial gastrocnemius, medial hamstring complex, anterior tibialis, and posterior tibialis.
   c. semimembranosus, semitendinosus, vastus medialis, and gluteus medius.
   d. Achilles' tendon, popliteus, and gluteus maximus/medius.

9. Key lengthening exercises via static or neuromuscular stretches for an individual with a foot/ankle impairment(s) include the

    a. medial gastrocnemius, medial hamstring complex, anterior tibialis, and gluteus medius.

    b. soleus/gastrocnemius, biceps femoris, and tensor fascia latae.

    c. semimembranosus, popliteus, and gluteus maximus/medius.

    d. Achilles' tendon, semitendinosus, vastus medialis, and posterior tibialis.

10. Key muscles to activate via isolated strengthening exercises or positional isometrics for an individual with a foot/ankle impairment(s) include the

    a. soleus/gastrocnemius, biceps femoris, and tensor fascia latae.

    b. toe flexors and intrinsic foot muscles, medial gastrocnemius, medial hamstring complex, anterior tibialis, and posterior tibialis.

    c. peroneus longus, peroneus brevis, and peroneus tertius.

    d. lateral gastrocnemius, vastus lateralis, and psoas major.

EXERCISE 12-4   **Practical Application**

INSTRUCTIONS: Design a corrective exercise program using the corrective exercise continuum for an individual with foot/ankle impairment.

ASSESSMENT FINDINGS:

- Static posture: Feet excessively pronated
- Overhead squat: Feet turn out (externally rotate) and flatten (evert)
- Single-leg squat: Feet flatten
- Gait: Excessive lower extremity pronation

PHASE	MODALITY	MUSCLE(S)/EXERCISE	ACUTE VARIABLES
Inhibit	Self-myofascial release		
Lengthen	Static stretching		
Activate	Isolated strengthening		
Integrate	Integrated dynamic movement		

CHAPTER 13

Corrective Strategies for Knee Impairments

EXERCISE 13-1   True/False

INSTRUCTIONS: Choose whether each statement is true or false.

1. The foot and ankle and the lumbo-pelvic-hip complex (LPHC) play a major role in knee impairment.

   True   False

2. The femur and the pelvis make up the sacroiliac joint.

   True   False

3. The sacrum and pelvis make up the iliofemoral joint.

   True   False

4. Patellar tendinopathy occurs when repeated stress is placed on the patellar tendon.

   True   False

5. Patellar tendinopathy is an injury common with athletes participating in jumping sports such as basketball, volleyball, or high or long jumping.

   True   False

6. Poor eccentric deceleration capabilities, overtraining, and playing on hard surfaces are all risk factors for patellar tendinopathy.

   True   False

7. Weakness in the hip abductor muscles, such as the gluteus medius, may result in synergistic dominance of the tensor fascia latae and consequently iliotibial band syndrome.

   True   False

8. When the patella is not properly aligned within the femoral trochlea, the stress per unit area on the patellar cartilage increases owing to a smaller contact area between the patella and the trochlea.

   True   False

9. Male athletes are at greater risk of ACL injury when compared with female athletes.

   True   **False**

10. Increased hip adduction motion in the frontal plane during athletic activities may place the athlete at increased risk of knee injury.

    True   **False**

11. If an individual does not have the capabilities to perform the tuck jump assessment, a basic gait analysis can also be performed, looking for overpronation of the foot and excessive knee valgus.

    True   **False**

12. To target ligament dominance deficits, the health and fitness professional should instruct the individual to use the knee as a frontal-plane hinge joint allowing abduction and adduction, not flexion and extension motions at the knee.

    True   **False**

13. The long jump and hold exercise allows the health and fitness professional to assess the individual's knee motion while he or she progresses through movements in the sagittal plane.

    True   **False**

14. One specific area that the health and fitness professional should focus on when training to prevent ACL injury risk is the correction of lower extremity valgus during jump landing tasks and cutting maneuvers.

    True   **False**

15. The health and fitness professional must be diligent in providing adequate feedback of correct technical performance (i.e., proper landing mechanics) to facilitate desirable neuromusculoskeletal alterations.

    True   **False**

EXERCISE 13-2   **Multiple Choice**

INSTRUCTIONS: Select the best answer from the choices given for each question.

1. Researchers have estimated health care costs to be approximately _____ annually for ACL injuries.
   a. $2.5 million
   b. $25 million
   c. $2.5 billion
   d. $25 billion

2. Risk factors for patellar tendinopathy include all of the following EXCEPT:
   a. knee valgus and varus.
   b. an increased Q-angle.
   c. 20 degrees of available ankle dorsiflexion.
   d. poor quadriceps and hamstring complex flexibility.

3. Inflammation and irritation of the distal portion of the iliotibial tendon as it rubs against the lateral femoral condyle is known as:
   a. iliotibial band syndrome (ITBS).
   b. patellar tendinopathy.
   c. patellofemoral syndrome.
   d. anterior cruciate ligament injury.

4. Abnormal tracking of the patella may be caused by all of the following EXCEPT:
   a. increased Q-angle.
   b. dynamic lower extremity malalignment.
   c. decreased strength of the hip musculature.
   d. static stretching before athletic activities.

5. Most noncontact ACL injuries occur when
   a. landing or decelerating on a single limb.
   b. jumping or accelerating on a single limb.
   c. sprinting in the sagittal plane.
   d. performing squatting motions with deep knee flexion.

6. Inflammation and irritation of the iliotibial band (ITB) may occur because of a lack of flexibility of the _____ _____ _____, which can result in an increase in tension on the ITB during the stance phase of running.
   a. pes anserine complex
   b. tensor fascia latae
   c. deep cervical flexors
   d. superficial erector spinae

7. _____ _____ could be used to target ligament dominance because this low-to-moderate-intensity jump movement does not go through deep knee flexion angles.
   a. Wall jumps
   b. Long jumps
   c. Box jumps
   d. 180-degree jumps

8. The _____ _____ is an integrated dynamic movement exercise to teach lower extremity control while the body is rotating in the transverse plane.
   a. wall jump
   b. long jump
   c. 180-degree jump
   d. tuck jump

9. What is the proper progression of jumping tasks from easiest to most difficult?
   a. Wall jumps → tuck jumps → long jumps → 180-degree jumps → single-leg hops → cutting maneuvers
   b. Tuck jumps → wall jumps → 180-degree jumps → long jumps → single-leg hops → cutting maneuvers
   c. Cutting maneuvers → 180-degree jumps → long jumps → tuck jumps → single-leg hops → wall jumps
   d. Long jumps → 180-degree jumps → cutting maneuvers → tuck jumps → single-leg hops → wall jumps

10. During competition, athletes may display _____ _____, a position of hip adduction and knee abduction that is the result of muscular contraction rather than ground reaction forces.
    a. active valgus
    b. plantar flexion
    c. active varus
    d. ankle inversion

EXERCISE 13-3 **Practical Application**

Design a corrective exercise program using the Corrective Exercise Continuum for an individual with knee impairment.

ASSESSMENT FINDINGS

- Static posture: feet pronated with tibial and femoral adduction and internal rotation
- Overhead squat: knees move inward
- Single-leg squat: knee moves inward
- Tuck jump: slight knee valgus and poor foot placement on landing

PHASE	MODALITY	MUSCLE(S)/EXERCISE	ACUTE VARIABLES
Inhibit	Self-myofascial release		
Lengthen	Static stretching		
Activate	Isolated strengthening		
Integrate	Integrated dynamic movement		

CHAPTER 14

Corrective Strategies for Lumbo-Pelvic-Hip Impairments

EXERCISE 14-1   True/False

INSTRUCTIONS: Choose whether each statement is true or false.

1. The lumbo-pelvic-hip complex has between 29 and 35 muscles that attach to the lumbar spine and pelvis.

   True   **False**

2. Many of the common injuries associated with the lumbo-pelvic-hip complex include low-back pain, sacroiliac joint dysfunction, and hamstring, quadriceps, and groin strains.

   True   **False**

3. Injuries that can stem from lumbo-pelvic-hip dysfunction include patellar tendinosis (jumper's knee), iliotibial band (IT band) tendonitis (runner's knee), and ACL tears.

   True   **False**

4. Compensation or dysfunctions in the lumbo-pelvic-hip complex rarely leads to dysfunction in the cervical-thoracic spine, ribs, shoulder, or upper extremity regions.

   True   **False**

5. If there is a lack of sagittal plane dorsiflexion at the ankle owing to an overactive or tight gastrocnemius and soleus, the lumbo-pelvic-hip complex may be forced to increase forward flexion of the trunk to alter the body's center of gravity to maintain balance.

   True   **False**

6. Lengthened and weak gastrocnemius, soleus, and hip flexor muscles produce the compensation of an excessive forward lean of the torso during squatting motions.

   True   **False**

7. As a compensatory mechanism for the underactivity and inability of the gluteus maximus to maintain an upright trunk position, the latissimus dorsi may become synergistically dominant (overactive or tight) to provide stability through the trunk, core, and pelvis.

   True　　**False**

8. The latissimus dorsi attaches to the pelvis and will posteriorly rotate the pelvis, which causes extension of the lumbar spine.

   True　　**False**

9. If the anterior tibialis and erector spinae are working at a submaximal level (underactive), the biceps femoris may become overactive to help maintain stabilization of the lumbo-pelvic-hip complex.

   True　　**False**

10. Increased hip or spinal flexion as a result of weakened gluteus maximus and erector spinae muscles can lead to excessive stress being placed on the low back, hamstring complex, and adductor magnus.

    True　　**False**

EXERCISE 14-2　**Practical Application**

INSTRUCTIONS: Design corrective exercise programs based on the individual's movement compensation illustrated in the images below.

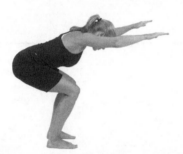

PHASE	MODALITY	MUSCLE(S)/EXERCISE	ACUTE VARIABLES
Inhibit	Self-myofascial release		
Lengthen	Static stretching		
Activate	Isolated strengthening		
Integrate	Integrated dynamic movement		

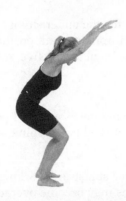

PHASE	MODALITY	MUSCLE(S)/EXERCISE	ACUTE VARIABLES
Inhibit	Self-myofascial release		
Lengthen	Static stretching		
Activate	Isolated strengthening		
Integrate	Integrated dynamic movement		

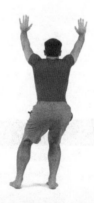

PHASE	MODALITY	MUSCLE(S)/EXERCISE	ACUTE VARIABLES
Inhibit	Self-myofascial release		
Lengthen	Static stretching		
Activate	Isolated strengthening		
Integrate	Integrated dynamic movement		

CHAPTER 15

Corrective Strategies for Shoulder, Elbow, and Wrist Impairments

---

EXERCISE 15-1 **Essential Vocabulary**

PURPOSE: The purpose of this exercise is to have an understanding of key terms used in Chapter 15.

INSTRUCTIONS: Match each term with its proper definition.

VOCABULARY WORDS

1. ___ Circumduction

2. ___ Dyskinesis

3. ___ De Quervain syndrome

DEFINITIONS

A. An inflammation or a tendinosis of the sheath or tunnel that surrounds two tendons that control movement of the thumb.

B. The circular movement of a limb.

C. An alteration in the normal position or motion of the scapula during coupled scapulohumeral movements.

EXERCISE 15-2 **True/False**

INSTRUCTIONS: Choose whether each statement is true or false.

1. Shoulder pain is reported to occur in up to 21% of the general population with 40% persisting for at least 1 year at an estimated annual cost of $39 billion.

   True   **False**

2. Traumatic shoulder dislocation is more prevalent than shoulder impingement syndrome.

True   False

3. Individuals with shoulder dislocations experience recurrent instability within 2 years and are at risk of developing glenohumeral osteoarthritis secondary to the increased motion at the glenohumeral joint.

True   False

4. The glenohumeral joint is a nonsynovial articulation between the head of the humerus and the glenoid of the scapula.

True   False

5. The static stabilizers of the glenohumeral joint include the glenoid labrum and the glenohumeral joint capsule, which consists of two major ligaments, the middle and inferior glenohumeral ligaments.

True   False

6. At midranges of shoulder motion, the glenohumeral ligaments are relatively lax, and the joint must rely heavily on the musculature that surrounds the joint for dynamic stability.

True   False

7. The rotator cuff is made up of the supraspinatus and subscapularis anteriorly with the infraspinatus, teres major, and cervical erector spinae posteriorly.

True   False

8. The deltoid and supraspinatus work together in a force-couple to control the humeral head in the frontal plane.

True   False

9. The infraspinatus and teres minor internally rotate the glenohumeral joint and decelerate the humerus during external rotation.

True   False

10. The main action of the subscapularis is medial (internal) rotation of the humerus while also being the primary stabilizer and humeral head depressor.

True   False

EXERCISE 15-3   Multiple Choice

INSTRUCTIONS: Select the best answer from the choices given for each question.

1. Tightness in the pectoralis minor will limit the effectiveness of the serratus anterior to
   a. upwardly rotate and posteriorly tilt the scapula.
   b. downwardly rotate and anteriorly tilt the scapula.
   c. upwardly rotate and posteriorly tilt the clavicle.
   d. downwardly rotate and anteriorly tilt the humerus.

2. The pectoralis minor plays an important role in scapula malposition as it can pull the scapula into a more
   a. protracted and anteriorly tilted position.
   b. retracted and superiorly tilted position.
   c. protracted and posteriorly tilted position.
   d. retracted and inferiorly tilted position.

3. Rotator cuff conditions such as strains, ruptures, and tendinopathies account for approximately
   a. 10 to 15% of shoulder injuries.
   b. 25 to 30% of shoulder injuries.
   c. 45 to 50% of shoulder injuries.
   d. 75 to 80% of shoulder injuries.

4. Injuries to the capsuloligamentous structures lead to deficits in the passive stabilizing structures of the shoulder such as the
   a. teres minor, teres major, serratus anterior, and subscapularis.
   b. anterior, posterior, or inferior glenohumeral ligaments and the glenoid labrum.
   c. anterior cruciate, medial cruciate, and posterior cruciate ligaments.
   d. calcaneofibular, anterior talofibular, and posterior talofibular ligaments.

5. A common diagnosis broadly defined as compression of the structures that run beneath the coracoacromial arch is known as:
   a. glenohumeral osteoarthritis.
   b. subacromial impingement syndrome.
   c. frozen shoulder.
   d. shoulder dislocation.

6. Subacromial impingement syndrome involves all of the impinged structures EXCEPT:
   a. supraspinatus and infraspinatus tendons.
   b. subacromial bursa.
   c. long head of the biceps tendon.
   d. medial head of the triceps tendon.

7. What joint is a hinge joint and is the primary joint responsible for elbow flexion and extension?
   a. Radioulnar joint
   b. Humeroradial joint
   c. Humeroulnar joint
   d. Glenohumeral joint

8. Which muscle is the primary flexor of the elbow?
   a. Brachialis
   b. Triceps brachii
   c. Pronator teres
   d. Anconeus

9. _____ is the most prevalent elbow disorder characterized by pain slightly distal to the lateral epicondyle.
   a. Medial epicondylitis
   b. Biceps tendinitis
   c. Lateral epicondylitis
   d. Olecranon bursitis

10. A combination of movements that extend the shoulder and elbow are most effective for lengthening the
   a. long head of the triceps.
   b. medial head of the triceps.
   c. long head of the biceps.
   d. short head of the triceps.

EXERCISE 15-4   Practical Application

INSTRUCTIONS: Design a corrective exercise program using the Corrective Exercise Continuum for an individual with shoulder impairment.

ASSESSMENT FINDINGS

- Static posture assessment: upper crossed syndrome
- Overhead squat assessment: arms fall forward
- Shoulder flexion wall test: low back arches and elbow flexes

PHASE	MODALITY	MUSCLE(S)/EXERCISE	ACUTE VARIABLES
Inhibit	Self-myofascial release		
Lengthen	Static stretching		
Activate	Isolated strengthening		
Integrate	Integrated dynamic movement		

CHAPTER 16

Corrective Strategies for Cervical Spine Impairments

EXERCISE 16-1   True/False

INSTRUCTIONS: Choose whether each statement is true or false.

1. According to a survey conducted by the National Institute of Health Statistics (NIHS), neck pain is the third most common type of pain for Americans.

    True   **False**

2. According to a survey conducted by the National Institute of Health Statistics (NIHS), women are three times more likely to experience neck pain.

    True   **False**

3. The neck muscle system is intimately related with reflex systems concerned with vestibular function, proprioceptive systems, stabilization of the head and eyes, postural orientation, and stability of the whole body.

    True   **False**

4. The cervical spine begins at the base of the skull and includes nine vertebrae (C1–C9).

    True   **False**

5. As an individual's head migrates forward, the pelvis reflexively rotates anteriorly to readjust his or her center of gravity; this is known as the pelvo-ocular reflex.

    True   **False**

6. The base of the skull and C1 (atlas) make up the atlanto-occipital joint.

    True   **False**

7. The atlas (C1) and axis (C2) make up the atlanto-odontoid joint and atlanto-axial joints

    True   **False**

8. The deep neck flexors are often overactive and synergistically dominate to maintain an upright cervical spine position as a result of underactivity and weakness of the upper trapezius, levator scapula, and sternocleidomastoid.

   True   False

9. At the thoracolumbar spine, low-back pain and sacroiliac joint dysfunction may be seen with various compensations in posture as a result of cervical spine dysfunction.

   True   False

10. According to a survey conducted by the National Institute of Health Statistics (NIHS), severe stress can increase the risk of neck pain by one and a half times.

    True   False

▌ EXERCISE 16-2   **Multiple Choice**

INSTRUCTIONS: Select the best answer from the choices given for each question.

1. A key static postural distortion syndrome to look for to determine potential movement dysfunction at the cervical spine is the
   a. upper crossed postural distortion syndrome.
   b. lower crossed postural distortion syndrome.
   c. pronation distortion syndrome.
   d. de quervain syndrome

2. Abnormal asymmetric shifting of the cervical spine (lateral flexion, translation, or rotation) is MOST likely caused by an overactive and underactive right and left
   a. sternocleidomastoid, scalenes, levator scapulae, and upper trapezius.
   b. longus coli, longus capitis, and cervical erector spinae.
   c. rhomboids, lower trapezius, and rotator cuff.
   d. teres minor, infraspinatus, supraspinatus, and subscapularis.

3. Shoulder elevation during the overhead squat assessment is potentially caused by underactivity of the
   a. sternocleidomastoid, levator scapulae, and upper trapezius.
   b. middle and lower trapezius, rhomboids, and rotator cuff.
   c. anterior deltoid, pectoralis major, and pectoralis minor.
   d. suboccipitals, scalenes, and serratus anterior.

4. Shoulder elevation during the overhead squat assessment is potentially caused by overactivity of the
   a. middle and lower trapezius, rhomboids, and rotator cuff.
   b. teres minor, infraspinatus, supraspinatus, and subscapularis.
   c. sternocleidomastoid, levator scapulae, and upper trapezius.
   d. suboccipitals, posterior deltoid, and serratus anterior.

5. All of the following are key regions to inhibit if a client's head protrudes forward during the assessment process EXCEPT:
   a. sternocleidomastoid.
   b. levator scapulae.
   c. upper trapezius.
   d. serratus anterior.

6. All of the following are key regions to activate if a client's head protrudes forward during the assessment process EXCEPT:
   a. lower trapezius.
   b. levator scapulae.
   c. deep cervical flexors.
   d. thoracic extensors.

7. Which of the following exercises would be MOST appropriate if a client's head protrudes forward during the assessment process?
   a. Ball combo I with chin tuck
   b. Squat to row
   c. Lateral dumbbell raise
   d. Standing dumbbell shoulder press

8. Which muscle is the MOST appropriate to inhibit if the chin rotates to the right during the assessment process?
   a. Infraspinatus (right side)
   b. Sternocleidomastoid (left side)
   c. Upper trapezius (right side)
   d. Teres minor (left side)

9. Which muscle is the MOST appropriate to lengthen if the head laterally flexes during the assessment process?
   a. Scalene (side of shift)
   b. Sternocleidomastoid (opposite side of shift)
   c. Upper trapezius (opposite side of shift)
   d. Longus coli (side of shift)

10. Which muscle is the MOST appropriate to activate through isolated strengthening if the head laterally flexes during the assessment process?
    a. Upper trapezius (same side of shift)
    b. Scalene (same side of shift)
    c. Rhomboid and lower trapezius (opposite side of shift)
    d. Sternocleidomastoid (opposite side of shift)

EXERCISE 16-3   Practical Application

Design a corrective exercise program based on the individual's movement compensation illustrated in the image below.

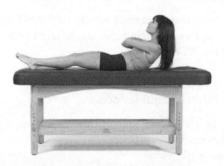

PHASE	MODALITY	MUSCLE(S)/EXERCISE	ACUTE VARIABLES
Inhibit	Self-myofascial release		
Lengthen	Static stretching		
Activate	Isolated strengthening		
Integrate	Integrated dynamic movement		

APPENDIX Answers to Exercises

CHAPTER 1   **EXERCISE 1-1**

1. F	3. A	5. E
2. D	4. B	6. C

EXERCISE 1-2

1. True
2. False—Today, approximately one third (33.8 percent) of adults are estimated to be obese.
3. True
4. False—Research suggests that musculoskeletal pain is more common now than it was 40 years ago. People are less active and are no longer spending as much of their free time engaged in physical activity producing more inactive and non-functional people.
5. True
6. True
7. True
8. False—Approximately 70 to 75 percent of ACL injuries are non-contact in nature.
9. True
10. True

EXERCISE 1-3

1. a	5. a	9. b
2. b	6. a	10. c
3. d	7. d	
4. c	8. a	

CHAPTER 2   **EXERCISE 2-1**

1. E	10. O	19. V
2. G	11. K	20. W
3. A	12. J	21. U
4. D	13. N	22. T
5. C	14. F	23. S
6. H	15. I	24. R
7. B	16. P	25. X
8. M	17. Z	26. Q
9. L	18. Y	

EXERCISE 2-2

1. Sagittal Plane
2. Frontal Plane
3. Transverse Plane
4. Pronation
5. Supination
6. Eccentric contraction
7. Isometric contraction
8. Concentric contraction

EXERCISE 2-3

1. a	6. c	11. d
2. b	7. d	12. a
3. c	8. a	13. c
4. d	9. c	14. a
5. a	10. a	15. b

CHAPTER 3

EXERCISE 3-1

1. G	5. F	9. I
2. D	6. H	10. C
3. A	7. B	
4. J	8. E	

EXERCISE 3-2

1. True
2. True
3. True
4. True
5. False—this is known as altered reciprocal inhibition
6. False—this is an example of altered reciprocal inhibition
7. True
8. True
9. True
10. False—these patterns of injury typically accompany an upper extremity movement impairment syndrome

EXERCISE 3-3

1. a	5. c	9. a
2. d	6. b	10. a
3. a	7. d	
4. d	8. b	

CHAPTER 4   EXERCISE 4-1

1. The three main pieces of information to ob[...] include one's physical readiness for activity, [...] medical history.

2. The Physical Activity Readiness Questionnai[...] termine if a person is ready to undertake lov[...] els. Furthermore, it aids in identifying peopl[...] not be appropriate or who may need further [...]

3. If an individual is sitting a large portion of th[...] longed periods of time. This, in turn, can lead [...] postural imbalances within the kinetic chain. [...] for prolonged periods of time, especially at a [...] the shoulders and head to fatigue under the constant influence of gravity. This often leads to a postural imbalance of rounding of the shoulders and head.

4. Construction workers and painters often work with their arms overhead for long periods of time. This may lead to possible shoulder soreness and tightness of the latissimus dorsi and weakness of the rotator cuff. This imbalance does not allow for proper shoulder motion and/or stabilization during activity.

5. Wearing shoes with a heel puts the ankle complex in a plantarflexion position for extended periods of time. This can lead to tightness in the gastrocnemius and soleus causing postural imbalance, such as over-pronation at the foot and ankle complex (flattening of the arch of the foot).

EXERCISE 4-2

1. True

2. False—By finding out what recreational activities and hobbies an individual performs, a health and fitness professional can better design a program to fit these needs.

3. True

4. True

5. True

6. True

7. True

8. False—It is estimated that more than 75 percent of the American adult population does not partake, on a daily basis, in 30 minutes of low-to-moderate physical activity.

9. False—It is *not* the role of a health and fitness professional to administer, prescribe or educate on the usage and effects of any of these medications.

10. True

EXERCISE 4-3

Potential "red flags" that may need to be considered when designing a corrective exercise program for this client include:

- **Extended periods of sitting:** This individual sits for extended periods of time primarily behind a computer which may cause tightness in the hip flexors, and a tendency for the shoulders and head to fatigue under the constant influence of gravity. This often leads to rounded shoulders and forward head posture.
- **Dress shoes with heel:** Wearing shoes with a heel puts the ankle complex in a plantarflexion position for extended periods of time. This can lead to tightness in the gastrocnemius and soleus causing postural imbalance, such as over-pronation at the foot and ankle complex.
- **Stress and Mental Anxiety:** Mental stress or anxiety can lead to a dysfunctional breathing pattern that can further lead to postural distortion and kinetic chain dysfunction.
- **Inactivity:** The individual's primary hobbies include reading and playing video games. These activities are relatively sedentary and it is quite possible this individual does not partake, on a daily basis, in 30 minutes of low-to-moderate physical activity. This lack of physical activity greatly increases the risk of chronic disease, in addition to a de-conditioned musculoskeletal system.
- **Intermittent low back pain:** This individual's low back pain may be caused by a several factors including extended periods of sitting, wearing dress shoes with an elevated heel, and overall inactivity leading to a de-conditioned musculoskeletal system and possible muscle imbalances.

CHAPTER 5

EXERCISE 5-1

1. E	4. C	7. D
2. A	5. I	8. F
3. G	6. B	9. H

EXERCISE 5-2

1. True
2. True
3. True
4. False—The assessment may not be able to specifically identify if a problem is structural (or biomechanical) in nature or if it is derived from the development of poor muscular recruitment patterns with resultant muscle imbalances.
5. True
6. False—The combination of tight and weak muscles can alter normal movement patterns.
7. True
8. True
9. True
10. True

EXERCISE 5-3

1. d	6. a	11. d
2. c	7. d	12. c
3. d	8. d	13. a
4. a	9. c	14. a
5. b	10. b	15. d

CHAPTER 6

EXERCISE 6-1

1. D   3. A   5. B
2. C   4. E

EXERCISE 6-2

1. True
2. True
3. True
4. True
5. False—Transitional movement assessments are assessments that involve movement without a change in one's base of support such as squatting, pressing, pushing, pulling, and balancing.
6. False—Dynamic movement assessments are assessments that involve movement with a change in one's base of support such as walking and jumping.
7. False—Knee valgus during the overhead squat test is influenced by decreased hip abductor and hip external rotation strength, increased hip adductor activity, and restricted ankle dorsiflexion.
8. True
9. True
10. True

EXERCISE 6-3

1. b   9. a   17. d
2. c   10. c   18. d
3. a   11. a   19. c
4. d   12. d   20. d
5. a   13. d   21. c
6. d   14. a   22. a
7. a   15. d   23. d
8. b   16. a   24. c

CHAPTER 7

EXERCISE 7-1

1. B   2. C   3. A

EXERCISE 7-2

1. True
2. True
3. True
4. False—In most normal subjects, passive ROM is slightly greater than active ROM.
5. True
6. True
7. False—Intratester reliability refers to the amount of agreement between goniometric values obtained by the same tester.
8. False—Intertester reliability refers to the amount of agreement between goniometric values obtained by different testers.

9. False—Validity of joint motion assessment reflects how closely the measurement represents the actual angle or total available range of motion.

10. False—Reliability refers to the amount of agreement between successive measurements.

EXERCISE 7-3

1. c	3. a
2. d	4. b

EXERCISE 7-4

1. a	10. c	19. a
2. b	11. d	20. b
3. d	12. b	21. d
4. b	13. d	22. c
5. b	14. a	23. a
6. a	15. b	24. c
7. c	16. b	25. d
8. a	17. d	26. c
9. d	18. a	

CHAPTER 8

EXERCISE 8-1

1. A	3. C	5. E
2. D	4. B	

EXERCISE 8-2

1. True

2. True

3. False—While other methods of evaluating muscle function exist that are more objective and reliable than manual muscle testing, such as isokinetic testing or hand-held dynamometry, manual muscle testing provides an opportunity to assess muscle function with low cost and difficulty.

4. True

5. True

6. True

7. True

8. False—The numerical grade of 3 represents a client who maintains good structural alignment and holds the end-range position against the assessor's pressure, which indicates a pure isometric contraction is present.

9. False—A numerical grade of 1 indicates little to no ability of the client to withstand or resist pressure from the assessor.

10. True

EXERCISE 8-3

1. d	8. c	15. a
2. b	9. b	16. c
3. a	10. a	17. b
4. a	11. d	18. a
5. b	12. a	19. a
6. c	13. c	20. d
7. a	14. c	

CHAPTER 9

EXERCISE 9-1

1. B	3. E	5. C
2. A	4. D	

EXERCISE 9-2

1. True
2. True
3. True
4. True
5. True
6. True
7. False—Increasing vasodilation, the tissue can receive adequate amounts of oxygen and nutrients as well as removal of waste bi-products (via blood) to facilitate tissue recovery and repair.
8. True
9. False—The autonomic nervous system's response to sustained pressure changes global muscle tonus as well as fluid dynamics to decrease viscosity and the tonus of the smooth muscle cells located in fascia.
10. False—Decreasing sympathetic tone reduces the prolonged faulty contraction of muscle tissue that can lead to the cumulative injury cycle.
11. False—One should begin using a softer foam roller, which offers less penetration into the soft tissue due to its increased compressibility
12. True
13. True
14. True
15. False—Anyone using SMR techniques should follow the same precautionary measures as those established for massage and/or myofascial release. SMR should be cautioned or avoided by people with congestive heart failure, kidney failure and/or any organ failure such as the liver and pancreas, bleeding disorders, and contagious skin conditions.

EXERCISE 9-3

1. c	5. c	9. a
2. a	6. b	10. b
3. a	7. a	
4. b	8. a	

EXERCISE 9-4

FREQUENCY	SETS	REPETITIONS	DURATION
Daily* (unless specified otherwise)	1	N/A	Hold tender spots for 30 to 90 seconds depending on intensity of application

CHAPTER 10

EXERCISE 10-1

1. A
2. C
3. B

EXERCISE 10-2

1. True
2. True
3. True
4. True
5. True
6. False—In general, it is thought that static stretching of 20–30 seconds causes an acute viscoelastic stress relaxation response allowing for an immediate increase in range of motion.
7. True
8. True
9. True
10. False—Stretching exercises are primarily used to increase the available range of motion (ROM) at a particular joint, specifically if the ROM at that joint is limited by tight neuromyofascial tissues. The scientific literature strongly supports the use of stretching exercises to achieve this goal.
11. False—Several researchers suggest that each joint and muscle group may respond differently to stretching protocols, thus each tissue to be stretched should be carefully evaluated, and the stretching protocol may need to be different for each range of motion limitation found.
12. True
13. True
14. False—The current evidence suggests that pre-exercise stretching does not have a significant impact on injury risk or rates although the effects of chronic, long-term stretching protocols tends to lead to decreased injury rates.
15. True
16. True
17. True
18. True

19. True

20. False—In a corrective exercise program, static stretching should only be applied to muscles that have been determined to be overactive/tight during the assessment.

21. False—Most of the current research has demonstrated that neuromuscular stretching is equally effective at increasing range of motion when compared to static stretching.

22. True

23. False—It is believed that the isometric contraction used during neuromuscular stretching decreases motor neuron excitability as a result of stimulation to the Golgi tendon organ and that this leads to autogenic inhibition resulting in decreased resistance to a change in length (or, ability to increase length of tissue).

24. True

25. True

26. True

27. True

28. True

29. True

30. True

EXERCISE 10-3

1. c	6. b	11. d
2. a	7. a	12. a
3. a	8. c	13. b
4. b	9. b	14. c
5. c	10. a	15. d

EXERCISE 10-4

A. Acute Variables for Static Stretching

FREQUENCY (PER WEEK)	SETS	REPETITIONS	DURATION OF EACH REPETITION
Daily (unless specified otherwise)	N/A	1-4	20-30 second hold 60 second hold for older patients (65 years +)

B. Acute Variables for Neuromuscular Stretching

FREQUENCY (PER WEEK)	SETS	REPETITIONS	DURATION OF EACH REPETITION
Daily (unless specified otherwise)	N/A	1-3	Contraction: 7 to 15 seconds Stretch: 20-30 seconds Intensity: submaximal, approximately 20-25% of maximal contraction

CHAPTER 11

EXERCISE 11-1

1. A	3. B	5. C
2. D	4. E	

EXERCISE 11-2

1. True
2. True
3. False—Isolated strengthening is a technique used to increase **intramuscular coordination** of specific muscles
4. True
5. True
6. True
7. False—Research has shown that the short-term use of unilateral and bilateral exercises is both effective at increasing performance measures and that unilateral exercise has a greater influence on unilateral performance.
8. True
9. False—Resistance training performed on unstable surfaces can be challenging and could be considered to assist in improvements in movement.
10. False—Integrated dynamic movement involves low load and controlled movement in ideal posture.

EXERCISE 11-3

1. b	6. d	11. b
2. c	7. c	12. b
3. a	8. b	13. a
4. d	9. a	14. a
5. a	10. a	15. a

CHAPTER 12

EXERCISE 12-1

1. D	4. C	7. H
2. A	5. F	8. G
3. E	6. B	9. I

EXERCISE 12-2

1. True
2. True
3. True
4. False—The subtalar joint consists of the talus and calcaneus.
5. True
6. True
7. False—The medial longitudinal arch is comprised of the calcaneus, talus, navicular, medial cuneiform, and first metatarsal.
8. True

9. True

10. False—The gastrocnemius complex, which consists of the gastrocnemius and soleus muscles, shares a common Achilles tendon that inserts on the base of the calcaneus.

EXERCISE 12-3

1. d	5. d	9. b
2. a	6. c	10. b
3. d	7. d	
4. a	8. a	

EXERCISE 12-4

PHASE	MODALITY	MUSCLE(S)/EXERCISE	ACUTE VARIABLES
Inhibit	Self-myofascial release	Lat. Gastrocnemius Peroneals Biceps femoris (short head)	Hold on tender area for 30 sec.
Lengthen	Static stretching	Gastrocnemius/soleus Biceps femoris (short head)	30-sec. hold
Activate	Isolated strengthening	Posterior tibialis Anterior tibialis Med. Hamstrings Med. Gastrocnemius	10-15 reps with 2-sec. isometric hold and 4-sec. eccentric
Integrate	Integrated dynamic movement	Single-leg Balance Reach Step Up to Balance	10-15 reps under control

CHAPTER 13

EXERCISE 13-1

1. True

2. False—The femur and the pelvis make up the iliofemoral joint.

3. False—The sacrum and pelvis make up the sacroiliac joint.

4. True

5. True

6. True

7. True

8. True

9. False—Female athletes are at greater risk of ACL injury, due to insufficient frontal plane control of the lower extremities.

10. True

11. True

12. False—To target ligament dominance deficits, the health and fitness professional should instruct individuals to use the knee as a single-plane (sagittal) hinge joint allowing flexion and extension, not valgus and varus motion at the knee.

13. True
14. True
15. True

EXERCISE 13-2

1. c	5. a	9. a
2. c	6. b	10. a
3. a	7. a	
4. d	8. c	

EXERCISE 13-3

This is one example of a corrective exercise program for the impairment of "knees move inward." However, whenever designing a corrective exercise program, the actual exercises used may be dependent on additional assessment findings and the individual's physical capabilities.

PHASE	MODALITY	MUSCLE(S)/EXERCISE	ACUTE VARIABLES
Inhibit	Self-myofascial release	Gastrocnemius/Soleus Adductors TFL/IT-band Biceps Femoris (short head)	Hold on tender area for 30 sec.
Lengthen	Static stretching	Lat. Gastrocnemius Adductors Tensor Fascia Latae Biceps Femoris	30-sec. hold
Activate	Isolated strengthening	Anterior Tibialis Posterior Tibialis Gluteus Medius Gluteus Maximus	10–15 reps with 2-sec. isometric hold and 4-sec. eccentric
Integrate	Integrated synamic movement	Jumping Progression: • Wall Jumps • Tuck Jumps • Long Jumps • 180-degree Jumps • Single-leg Hops • Cutting Maneuvers	10–15 reps under control

CHAPTER 14

EXERCISE 14-1

1. True
2. True
3. True
4. False—The body is an interconnected chain and compensation or dysfunction in the LPHC region can lead to dysfunctions in other areas of the body. Moving above the LPHC, common injuries are often seen in the cervical-thoracic spine, ribs, shoulder and upper extremity regions which can stem from dysfunction in the LPHC.

5. True

6. False—The under activity of the erector spinae and gluteus maximus to maintain an upright trunk position produce the compensation of an excessive forward lean. The gastrocnemius, soleus, and hip flexor muscles are typically tight and overactive when an individual exhibits an excessive forward lean during squatting motions.

7. True

8. False—The latissimus dorsi attaches to the pelvis and will anteriorly rotate the pelvis which causes extension of the lumbar spine.

9. True

10. True

EXERCISE 14-2

Below is one example of a corrective exercise program for the impairment of "excessive forward lean." However, whenever designing a corrective exercise program, the actual exercises used may be dependent on additional assessment findings and the individual's physical capabilities.

PHASE	MODALITY	MUSCLE(S)/EXERCISE	ACUTE VARIABLES
Inhibit	Self-myofascial release	Gastrocnemius/soleus Hip flexor complex	Hold on tender area for 30-sec
Lengthen	Static stretching	Gastrocnemius/soleus Hip flexor complex Abdominal complex	30-sec hold
Activate	Isolated strengthening	Anterior tibialis Gluteus maximus Erector spinae Core stabilizers	10–15 reps with 2-sec isometric hold and 4-sec eccentric
Integrate	Integrated dynamic movement	Ball wall squat with overhead press	10–15 reps under control

Below is one example of a corrective exercise program for the impairment of "low back rounds." However, whenever designing a corrective exercise program, the actual exercises used may be dependent on additional assessment findings and the individual's physical capabilities.

PHASE	MODALITY	MUSCLE(S)/ EXERCISE	ACUTE VARIABLES
Inhibit	Self-myofascial release	Hamstrings Adductor magnus	Hold on tender area for 30-sec
Lengthen	Static stretching	Hamstrings Adductor magnus Abdominal complex	30-sec hold
Activate	Isolated strength-ening	Gluteus maximus Hip flexors Erector spinae	10–15 reps with 2-sec isometric hold and 4-sec eccentric
Integrate	Integrated dynamic movement	Ball wall squat with overhead press	10–15 reps under control

Below is one example of a corrective exercise program for the impairment of "asymmetrical weight shift." However, whenever designing a corrective exercise program, the actual exercises used may be dependent on additional assessment findings and the individual's physical capabilities.

PHASE	MODALITY	MUSCLE(S)/EXERCISE	ACUTE VARIABLES
Inhibit	Self-myofascial release	Adductors,TFL/IT band (right side) Piriformis, Biceps femoris (left side)	Hold on tender area for 30-sec
Lengthen	Static stretching	Adductors, Tensor fascia latae (right side) Piriformis Biceps femoris (left side)	30-sec hold
Activate	Isolated strengthening	Gluteus medius (right side) Adductors (left side)	10–15 reps with 2-sec isometric hold and 4-sec eccentric
Integrate	Integrated dynamic movement	Ball wall squat to overhead press	10–15 reps under control

CHAPTER 15

EXERCISE 15-1

1. B
2. C
3. A

EXERCISE 15-2

1. True
2. False—Shoulder impingement is the most prevalent diagnosis accounting for 40-65% of reported shoulder pain while traumatic shoulder dislocations account for an additional 15-25% of shoulder pain.
3. True
4. False—The glenohumeral joint is a ball and socket articulation between the head of the humerus and the glenoid of the scapula.
5. True
6. True
7. False—The rotator cuff is made up of the supraspinatus and subscapularis anteriorly with the infraspinatus, teres minor posteriorly.
8. True
9. False—The infraspinatus and teres minor externally rotate the glenohumeral joint and decelerate the humerus during internal rotation.
10. True

EXERCISE 15-3

1. a	5. b	9. c
2. a	6. d	10. c
3. d	7. c	
4. b	8. a	

EXERCISE 15-4

Below is one example of a corrective exercise program for shoulder impairment in which the client displays multiple movement impairments. However, whenever designing a corrective exercise program, the actual exercises used may be dependent on additional assessment findings and the individual's physical capabilities.

PHASE	MODALITY	MUSCLE(S)/EXERCISE	ACUTE VARIABLES
Inhibit	Self-myofascial release	Latissimus dorsi Thoracic spine	Hold on tender area for 30 sec.
Lengthen	Static stretching	Latissimus dorsi Pectoralis major Erector spinae Biceps brachii	30-sec. hold
Activate	Isolated strengthening	Rotator cuff Rhomboids Middle & lower trapezius Core stabilizers	10–15 reps with 2-sec. isometric hold and 4-sec. eccentric
Integrate	Integrated dynamic movement	Squat to row	10–15 reps under control

CHAPTER 16

EXERCISE 16-1

1. True
2. True
3. True
4. False—The cervical spine begins at the base of the skull and includes seven vertebrae (C1-C7).
5. True
6. True
7. True
8. False—As a compensatory mechanism for the underactivity and inability of the deep neck flexors and cervical erector spinae to maintain an upright cervical spine position, the upper trapezius, levator scapula, sternocleidomastoid and pectoralis become synergistically dominant (overactive) in order to provide stability through the core and shoulder girdle complex
9. True
10. True

EXERCISE 16-2

1. a
2. a
3. b
4. c
5. d
6. b
7. a
8. b
9. a
10. c

EXERCISE 16-3

Below is one example of a corrective exercise program for the impairment of a "forward head" posture. However, whenever designing a corrective exercise program, the actual exercises used may be dependent on additional assessment findings and the individual's physical capabilities.

PHASE	MODALITY	MUSCLE(S)/EXERCISE	ACUTE VARIABLES
Inhibit	Self-myofascial release	Thoracic spine Sternocleidomastoid Levator scapulae Upper trapezius	Hold on tender area for 30 seconds
Lengthen	Static stretching	Sternocleidomastoid Levator scapulae Upper trapezius	30-second hold
Activate	Isolated strengthening	Deep cervical flexors Cervical erector spinae Lower trapezius	10–15 reps with 2-second isometric hold and 4-second eccentric
Integrate	Integrated dynamic movement	Ball combo 1 w/ cervical retraction	10–15 reps under control